PREVENTION AND CONTROL OF PAIN IN CHILDREN

A manual for health professionals based on the
findings of a workshop of the Royal College of
Paediatrics and Child Health, London, chaired by

David Southall

Foundation Professor of Paediatrics, Keele University
Consultant Paediatrician, North Staffordshire Hospital
Honorary Director, Child Advocacy International

BMJ
Publishing
Group

First published in 1997
by the BMJ Publishing Group, BMA House,
Tavistock Square, London WC1H 9JR

British Library Cataloguing in Publication Data

A catalogue record for this book is available
from the British Library

ISBN 0–7279–1178–3

Typeset, printed and bound in Great Britain by
Latimer Trend and Company Ltd, Plymouth

Contents

Contributors

David Burge Honorary Secretary, British Association of Paediatric Surgeons

Susan Burr Adviser in Paediatric Nursing to the Royal College of Nursing

Ann Goldman Consultant in Palliative Care, Great Ormond Street Hospital for Children, London

Noelle Llewellyn Chair of the Royal College of Nursing (RCN) Paediatric Pain Interest Group; Clinical nurse specialist, Pain Control Team, Great Ormond Street Hospital for Children, London

Adrian Lloyd-Thomas Consultant Anaesthetist; Director, Pain Control Team, Great Ormond Street Hospital for Children, London; representing the Royal College of Anaesthetists

Karen Lovatt Clinical Pharmacist, North Staffordshire Hospital

Harvey Marcovitch Consultant Paediatrician and Honorary Editor, the Royal College of Paediatrics and Child Health

Neil McIntosh Professor of Child Life and Health, University of Edinburgh

Neil Morton Consultant in Paediatric Anaesthesia and Intensive Care, Royal Hospital for Sick Children, Glasgow; representing the Association of Paediatric Anaesthetists of Great Britain and Ireland

Barbara Phillips Consultant Paediatrician in Accident and Emergency, Alder Hey Children's Hospital, Liverpool

David Southall Professor of Paediatrics, North Staffordshire Hospital, Keele University
(*Chairman of Working Party*)

Martin Ward Platt Consultant Paediatrician, Royal Victoria Infirmary, Newcastle-upon-Tyne

Special thanks to:
Martin Becker Consultant Paediatrician, Hinchingbrooke Hospital

Imti Choonara Senior Lecturer in Paediatric Clinical Pharmacology, Alder Hey Children's Hospital

Peter Crowle Consultant Paediatrician, Norfolk and Norwich NHS Trust

Peter Fleming Professor of Infant Health and Developmental Physiology, Institute of Child Health, Bristol

Chrissi Hart Consultant Clinical Psychologist, Special Interest Group, British Psychological Society

Angela O'Higgins Clinical Nurse Specialist, Paediatric Intensive Care Unit, North Staffordshire Hospital

Charlotte Howell Consultant Paediatric Anaesthetist, North Staffordshire Hospital

Anne Hunt Nurse researcher, Royal College of Nursing Institute

Andrew Magnay Paediatric Intensivist and Director of Paediatric Intensive Care Unit, North Staffordshire Hospital

Tony Nunn Director of Pharmacy, Alder Hey Children's Hospital

Heather MacKinnon Consultant Paediatrician, The Whittington Hospital

Ginny McGivern Nurse Coordinator, Complementary Therapy Unit, Queen's Medical Centre, Nottingham

Helen McGowan The Paediatric Macmillan Team, Alder Hey Children's Hospital

Lorna McKenna Medical Secretary, North Staffordshire Hospital

D. E. Murfin Family Practitioner, Brynteg Surgery, Dyfed

Barry Pizer Consultant in Paediatric Oncology, Alder Hey Children's Hospital

Valerie Rigby The Paediatric Macmillan Team, Alder Hey Children's Hospital

Martin Samuels Senior Lecturer in Paediatrics, North Staffordshire Hospital

Paul Stallard Clinical Psychologist, Special interest group for children and young people, British Psychological Society

Terence Stephenson Professor of Child Health, Queen's Medical Centre, Nottingham

Benjamin Tura Research Assistant, North Staffordshire Hospital

Kate Verrier Jones Laura Ashley Senior Lecturer in Paediatric Nephrology, Cardiff Royal Infirmary

Janet Vickers The Paediatric Macmillan Team, Alder Hey Children's Hospital

Kathy Wilkinson Consultant Anaesthetist, Norfolk and Norwich NHS Trust

The doses of drugs listed in this book are to the best of our belief correct at the time of going to press. However, they should always be checked with the *British National Formulary*, a childrens' hospital formulary, or a pharmacist experienced in prescribing for children.

Foreword

An ability to prevent and, when this fails, to treat pain is essential for all doctors, nurses, and health professionals who care for sick or injured children. It is not an easy subject. The control of pain often requires powerful drugs with side effects, some of which can be fatal if not adequately identified and managed. The use of some analgesics, particularly the powerful opioid or sedative drugs, requires the highest level of training in airway management and other aspects of resuscitation. Unfortunately, an alternative approach, especially if one is insecure about one's skills in these areas, is to withhold or underprescribe such drugs. In infants in particular, who cry a lot anyway, this might not be noticed. Some children in pain may also respond by becoming quiet and withdrawn. A lack of recognition of pain can therefore be a successful way of avoiding the issue. There are also other excuses put forward for not using probably the most valuable of the pain-relieving drugs: the opioids. Excuses include the overestimated dangers of inducing dependence. This and other concerns are widely promoted in some countries and have led to a moratorium on the use of opioids in children. This is particularly worrying when such drugs can be invaluable in treating long term pain associated with such conditions as cancer or sickle cell disease.

The adequate control of pain in children requires a highly skilled approach encompassing the needs of the whole child by the most highly trained and experienced of healthcare professionals. Unfortunately, this is not always the case and many widely practised painful procedures on children (for example, intubation and venous cannulation) are often undertaken by the most junior of staff.

Since pain control involves so many different disciplines it is important that a team approach is adopted to its management. The establishment of pain control services within hospitals and community health centres is recommended.

This manual identifies a number of areas in which much more research is needed to optimise the control of pain in children. An example of this is venous cannulation which surely requires us to find better ways of helping the many children who need this procedure. We hope that paediatricians, nurses, family doctors, researchers, pharmacists, psychologists and all involved in managing this difficult but central aspect of care will look to new developments which will minimise the suffering of ill or injured children.

David Southall
January 1997

Glossary

The following units are used in the expression of drug dosages in this book:

h	hour
min	minute
s	second
/24 h	per 24 hours
/h	per hour
/min	per minute
kg	kilogram
g	gram
mg	milligram
l	litre
ml	millilitre

The doses of drugs listed in this book are to the best of our belief correct at the time of going to press. However, they should always be checked with the *British National Formulary*, a childrens' hospital formulary, or a pharmacist experienced in prescribing for children.

1 General concepts and recommendations

Before considering in detail strategies for the prevention and control of pain in children, it is worth outlining some broad concepts and recommendations.

CONCEPTS IN PAIN CONTROL

It is ethically wrong to allow an infant or older child to suffer uncontrolled pain. Every child deserves to have, and it is the duty of healthcare professionals to provide, adequate and safe pain control. Uncontrolled pain has adverse effects on cardiovascular, respiratory, immunological and metabolic processes, as well as long term psychological effects that are not fully quantified but likely to be harmful.

Children, especially preterm neonates and non-verbal children, are generally undertreated for pain,[1] receiving fewer, smaller doses of opioid drugs than are given to adults and, instead, being given more minor analgesics. Reasons for this include: fear of harmful side effects; belief that children do not feel pain as do adults; fear of causing addiction; fear of masking clinical signs and symptoms; the child's fear of receiving injections; and lack of communication between anaesthetists, surgeons, nursing staff and parents.

> *"Pain intrinsically is subjective and in order to be treated its presence must be communicated: pain cannot be palpated, weighed or measured. Trust and a common language are necessary for effective communication."*[2]

RECOMMENDATIONS FOR PAIN MANAGEMENT

Pain control should be a central concern of all healthcare professionals,[3] and each children's unit should have a specific pain

1

control service. The team providing the service should ideally comprise those individuals listed in Box 1.1, and function as outlined in Box 1.2.

Box 1.1—Ideal composition of a children's unit pain control service

- One or more clinical nurse specialists
- A paediatrician
- An anaesthetist with an interest in treating children
- A surgeon
- An accident and emergency specialist
- A child psychologist
- A clinical pharmacist
- A physiotherapist
- Hospital play specialists

Box 1.2—Activities of a pain control team

- Good communication between team members, on the principle of shared care and shared responsibility
- Setting of practical standards
- Establishment of "evidence-based" guidelines for pain management, updated regularly
- Audit of effectiveness, complications and patient satisfaction
- Training and education of staff, parents and children
- Establishment of strategies for the control of acute and chronic pain

---

The role of the pain control team is to develop a specific expertise relevant to the needs of their own unit, and to share this expertise when policies need to be established or reviewed.

A pain control service should probably include a smaller team responsible for the day to day management of pain in different areas of the hospital. The executive team could be led by a senior nurse specialist and paediatric anaesthetist.

Although a multidisciplinary approach is vital to the achievement of effective pain control, it is invariably nurses who will coordinate and implement the pain control protocols and identify the need for changes in care. This means they must be trained in pain assessment and pain management.

Individual and anticipatory care

Pain control plans should be individual to the child and to his or her family, and prepared in collaboration with them. For example, healthcare professionals should be aware of and respect cultural beliefs that relate to the meaning and control of pain. The ability to control pain should not be overstated to the child or parents—the aim is to achieve good control and complete pain relief may not be attainable. Parents should be informed about the pain relief that will be given to their child to make his or her stay in hospital as comfortable as possible, as set out in *The Patient's Charter*.[4]

When beginning a course of treatment for pain it is important never to assume that it will be short lived. Pain control must be of high quality from the onset, with an emphasis on preventive measures.

Attempts should always be made to anticipate and prevent pain rather than trying to relieve it when it is established. "As required" regimens should be avoided, and analgesics should be used in regular and adequate doses. It is important to ask for and value the child's judgement concerning the adequacy of pain relief provided. It is essential that the differences between acute and chronic pain are understood in terms of both assessment and management (for example, some of the non-pharmacological interventions are more effective with acute pain—see later.)

Non-pharmacological as well as pharmacological approaches can be valuable,[5] especially in chronic pain, remembering that the former are adjuvants, not substitutes. Some children who appear compliant with non-pharmacological approaches may be suffering in silence because they want to please or fear an injection.

Routes of administration of pain relief

There is little place for intramuscular pain relief, particularly as a repeated treatment. Many children would rather suffer their pain than receive intramuscular analgesia. However, when venous access is impossible, and where finding a vein would itself add to the child's suffering, a single intramuscular injection may be appropriate. Routes of administration of analgesics should be discussed with the child and parents. When using rectally administered drugs, attempts should be made, whenever possible, to obtain verbal consent from parents and child.

Fasting

Fasting guidelines (Box 1.3) need to be observed before all procedures involving sedation or powerful analgesia, although rigid routines should be avoided.

Box 1.3—Guidelines on fasting children before sedation or strong analgesia

- Food/milk/formula feed: nothing for 6 h
- Breast milk: nothing for 4 h
- Clear fluids: stop for 2–3 h before sedation or general anaesthesia
- If in doubt about the starvation time give only clear fluids (water, dextrose, diluted clear fruit juice (no particulate matter), other soft drinks)

Some hospital protocols stipulate "nothing from 12 midnight", with no regard to the number of hours the child is fasted. It is uncomfortable and potentially dangerous to fast children for prolonged periods, particularly young infants. The normal young child has a relative inability to maintain normoglycaemia during even 6–12 h without food,[6] and the maturing brains of young children also have an increased sensitivity to hypoglycaemia.[7] Nothing for 6 h should not mean nothing for 12 h when, for example, an operation is performed at noon and the child has been fasted since midnight.

Communication

It is difficult to know when it is best for parents to inform a child about a forthcoming medical or surgical procedure that will cause pain or discomfort. Generally, the younger the child the shorter should be the interval.

Healthcare professionals working with children should try to learn and practise verbal and non-verbal communication strategies, appropriate to children at various developmental stages, that may help the management of acute and chronic pain. For example:

- Find something positive to say about an aspect of the child's physical state
- Give a message that the child can be helpful or can master something in this situation, for example, allow them to choose how they will lie or where their mother will sit
- Use a distraction approach: speak in terms of going home, or playing after a painful procedure is over
- Use language that implies things will change, will get better and that there is a future, although for children with terminal illness this advice may have to be modified
- Accept some crying or shouting, which can be a form of distraction for the child.

If a conscious child has to be restrained for a procedure, kind but firm restraint must be exerted by a person (ideally a parent) or persons and not by devices such as straitjackets or the tying down of limbs. For inpatient care a comfortable bed for the parent next to the child should be offered. In selected cases it may be appropriate for parent and child to sleep together in the same bed. A majority of young children sleep with their parents when they are ill at home[8] and there is increasing evidence that it may have beneficial effects on the child.[9]

More ill children, particularly those with long term illnesses, are being cared for in the community. The information in this manual relates to children in all settings, including the home where their treatment may be supervised by paediatric community nurses. When a child needs pain control at home, the family doctor must be given detailed advice so that he or she can provide appropriate support for the child, family and healthcare team.

It may be difficult to assess pain and to ensure the adequacy of its control in children with developmental impairments. Research is needed into this important problem.

DEVELOPING A PAIN CONTROL SERVICE FOR CHILDREN

There are many new approaches to the control of children's pain, and these have great potential to help our young patients. However, change can be threatening for those concerned and it is vital that new practices in paediatric pain management are introduced in a logical, structured way, so that all those involved gain maximum benefit. Ways in which this can be achieved include the use of audit, standard setting and clinical guidelines.

Audit

Provision of pain relief is an indicator of the quality of care provided for children in hospital.[10] The use of audit to monitor practice in pain relief can provide a structure for future change and a means to reflect on change that has already occurred, while audit of particular areas of practice can provide a basis for refining care. Improvements identified in the quality of pain relief provided can be balanced against less desirable effects, such as nausea and vomiting following the use of patient controlled analgesia. In addition, a crucial element of a paediatric pain control service is the cost:benefit ratio of pain relief procedures. Use of a local

5

anaesthetic cream before giving injections, for example, is less expensive than time and energy otherwise spent in restraining children.

Standard setting

All experienced healthcare professionals have standards that reflect what they consider to be good, bad or indifferent practice. Formal standard setting enables individuals to agree a level of achievement for their clinical area of practice. Standard setting also enables those involved to identify what structures are required to achieve the agreed standards, how they will be achieved and what the results will be. Standard setting is an integral part of providing a high quality service.

Clinical guidelines

Clinical guidelines provide a link between academic research and everyday practice. They provide a means to support practice with evidence and to explore the options available in a given situation. The Department of Health in the UK has suggested that evidence-based guidelines are made part of purchaser/provider contracts within the National Health Service. With many innovative analgesic interventions now available, clinical guidelines can provide a framework upon which to base care, and information to which doctors and nurses can usefully refer.

In pain relief as in any other sphere, doctors and nurses should undertake only those duties that are within their area of professional competence and for which they have been properly trained.

PRESCRIBING FOR CHILDREN

In childhood, dosages are generally adjusted for weight until 50 kg, or puberty has been reached.

Prescriptions should be written according to guidelines outlined in the *British National Formulary*. Inclusion of age is a legal requirement in the case of "prescription only" medicines for children under 12 years of age but it is preferable to state the age on all prescriptions written for children. It is particularly important to state the strengths of capsules or tablets. When taken over a long period sugar free tablets and liquid medicines should be used whenever possible. When a prescription for a liquid oral preparation is written and the dose ordered is smaller than 5 ml the preparation will no longer be diluted, instead an oral syringe will be supplied.

In hospitals the appropriate prescription sheet must be used. Administration of medicines in hospital without a doctor's prescription must be according to the written protocols agreed by the professions and approved by the Trust.

The potential for medication error must be recognised. A multidisciplinary team must consider local practices and take steps to reduce the potential for error.

Parents should be advised not to add any medicines to the contents of an infant feeding bottle since the drug may react with the milk or other liquid in it.

Calculation by body weight in the obese child may result in higher doses being administered than are necessary. In such cases doses should be calculated from an ideal weight related to height and age.

Prescription of controlled drugs (see *British National Formulary*)

Orders for controlled drugs subject to prescription requirements in the community and for outpatients must be signed and dated by the prescriber and specify the prescriber's address. The prescription must always be stated in the prescriber's own handwriting in ink or otherwise so as to be indelible:

- The name and address of the patient
- In the case of a preparation, the form and where appropriate the strength of the preparation
- The total quantity of the preparation, or the number of dose units, in both words and figures
- The dose.

A prescription may order a controlled drug to be dispensed by instalments; the amount of the instalments and the intervals to be observed must be specified. Prescriptions ordering "repeats" on the same form are not permitted.

It is an offence for a doctor to issue an incomplete prescription and a pharmacist is not allowed to dispense a controlled drug unless all the information required by law is given on the prescription. Failure to comply with the regulations concerning the writing of prescriptions will result in inconvenience to patients and delay in supplying the necessary medicine.

The administration of sedative and analgesic drugs to children

In preparing a single dose or infusion, it is essential that two qualified members of the nursing and/or medical staff check the prescription, dose, formulation, dilution and administration to the patient of all drugs and in particular opioids. All parenterally given

7

agents should be regarded as high risk since errors may produce immediate adverse or even fatal effects.

This is particularly important, when, for example, morphine is being administered to an infant or young child. The original ampoule of morphine usually contains 10 mg in 1 ml (that is 10,000 microgram in 1 ml). Dilution of this powerful solution can be potentially dangerous if great care is not taken. We recommend that hospital pharmacies prepare or obtain specially made up solutions of morphine for use in infants and young children (perhaps 1 mg in 1 ml).

This manual does not address the management of children with repeated and unexplained headaches or abdominal pain.

REFERENCES

1 Schechter NL. The undertreatment of pain in children: an overview. *Pediatr Clin North Am* 1989;**36**:781–94.
2 Shapiro BS, Cohen DE, Howe CJ. Patient-controlled analgesia for sickle-cell related pain. *J Pain Symptom Man* 1993;**8**:22–8.
3 Shapiro BS. The management of pain in sickle cell disease. *Pediatr Clin North Am* 1989;**36**:1029–45.
4 *The Patient's Charter: services for children and young people*. Department of Health, London 1996.
5 McGrath PJ, Craig KD. Developmental and psychological factors in children's pain. *Pediatr Clin North Am* 1989;**36**:823–36.
6 Kelnar CJH. Hypoglycaemia in children undergoing adenotonsillectomy. *BMJ* 1976;**1**:751–2.
7 Haworth JC, Godin FJ. Idiopathic spontaneous hypoglycaemia in children. *Pediatrics* 1960;**25**:748–65.
8 Southall DP, Tura B, Morris J. Cosleeping for ill children at home and in hospital. In preparation.
9 McKenna J. Infant-parent co-sleeping in an evolutionary perspective— implications for understanding infant sleep development and the sudden infant death syndrome. *Sleep* 1993;**16**:263–82.
10 Audit Commission. *Children first—a study of hospital services*. London: HMSO, 1993.

2 Assessment of pain

In 1987 Wong and Baker[1] described the QUESTT approach to pain assessment (Box 2.1). We summarise in this chapter some approaches to the assessment of pain that may be of clinical value in children's units.

> **Box 2.1—The QUESTT approach to assessing pain in children**
>
> - Question the child
> - Use pain rating scales
> - Evaluate behavioural and physiological changes
> - Secure the parents' involvement
> - Take the cause of pain into account
> - Take action and evaluate the results

PROBLEMS WITH ASSESSMENT OF PAIN

Assessing the pain experienced by a child can be difficult, especially for inexperienced doctors and nurses. It is necessary to differentiate anxiety from pain, and be alert for covert suffering. An uncomplaining, silent child who lies still and rigid after an abdominal operation, scoring zero for pain at rest, may seem like the ideal patient to inexperienced staff. However, the child may be terrified to move in case it hurts, and may not complain for fear of an intramuscular injection.

Both parents and professionals may underestimate or overestimate the severity of pain in children,[2] and it is important to recognise that pre-verbal and non-verbal children (for example, those with learning difficulties or with sensory handicap) may be unable adequately to express their need for pain control.

Equally, an holistic approach to the child will reduce the risk of staff focusing on pain and its control to the exclusion of all else. For example, the restless child with cramping lower abdominal discomfort may have urinary retention and a full bladder, not wound pain.

METHODS FOR ASSESSING PAIN

The main methods of pain assessment are listed in Box 2.2, and will be discussed in turn.

Box 2.2—Methods for assessing pain in children

- Inference
- Discussion
- Self report scale
- Observation of behaviour
- Observation of physiological measures ± behavioural changes
- Keeping a diary

Inference

Doctors and nurses experienced in the type, severity and extent of injury or illness present can predict how bad the pain is likely to be and how long it might last. It is well established that experienced paediatric nurses are better at this than trainees and that parents can be better than nurses.[3]

Discussion

Discussion may be directly with the child or through the parents. Questions to ask are: Does anything hurt? Where does it hurt? What does it feel like? Body charts may help the child describe the site of the pain.

You can ask the child: Do you want me to do something to help? What makes the pain better or worse?

And ask the parents: Do you think we need to do something to relieve the pain?

More detailed questions may be appropriate, depending on the circumstances.

Cognitive, physiological, sensory, behavioural, affective, sociocultural and environmental factors all affect pain assessment. A good clinician or nurse uses knowledge of the child's age, social circumstances and cultural background to judge that particular child's needs. Is the child exhibiting behavioural, physiological or emotional evidence of pain and, if so, how severe is it? What intervention is appropriate to try to control the pain? Having intervened, the healthcare professional assesses whether the intervention is adequate and intervenes further if necessary. Staff may almost unconsciously compare a child with previous children they have cared for at, say, a certain stage after an operation, to judge whether he or she is following the anticipated path to recovery. Measurements with pain scales or scores should be regarded as an aid to this more complex holistic assessment process.

Remember that children need opportunities to talk about their pain control. In a busy ward this may be difficult, and some children may not like to disturb staff.

Self report scales

Available scales for the self reporting of pain in children are listed in Appendix A. Selection of an assessment scale should be based on:

- The age of the child
- His or her cognitive ability
- The time available for education about the scale
- The knowledge of nursing staff about the scale
- The preference of children who have used the different scales in the past.

It is better to use one or two scales regularly and know them well, rather than several scales infrequently. Scales selected should be simple, clear and easy to use. Self report scales[4-10] provide a subjective, quantitative measure of pain. They are generally considered suitable only for children over 4 years of age, as they all rely to some extent on the child having some idea of relative size or number. Many researchers consider self reporting to be the "gold standard" for the measurement of pain, but remember that the consequences of stating that he or she has pain may influence a child's responses; for example, a child may claim to have less pain if he or she fears a delay in going home from the hospital.

Observation of behaviour

Observations by the nurse caring for the child provide a basic start to the assessment of pain. For example, she can record:

- What is the child's conscious state? *Asleep/awake*. Proceed only if awake
- Is the child crying? *No/yes*

- What is the child's posture? *Relaxed/tense*
- What is the facial expression? *Neutral or happy/distressed*
- What is the response to questions? *Positive when talked to/ negative or non-responsive.*

Ideally, parents should collaborate in these observations of their child's behaviour. However, they are not specific and more information can be provided by using behavioural scales (Appendix B).[11–14] These scales attempt to equate vocalisations, motor responses, body posture, behavioural state and sleep with the presence or absence of pain. Some focus on specific behaviours such as facial expression, and others on broad-band behaviours.

It is important to recognise the limitations of behavioural scales in the assessment of pain. For example, behavioural patterns are age determined. Behavioural scales also measure the child's most vigorous response, and therefore generally fail to recognise the child whose behavioural patterns are diminished as a result of extreme or, particularly, long standing (chronic) pain. It is also generally felt that behavioural scales are less sensitive than self report scales to "slight" changes in pain levels.[15]

Observation of physiological measures ± behavioural changes

Cardiovascular and respiratory responses are generally monitored routinely during a hospital stay, but the contribution of these observations to pain assessment is debatable. The body's global, non-specific response to a painful stimulus may occur in other circumstances; and a child who is acutely ill may manifest changes in his or her vital signs as a result of the disease or illness process or as a result of injury. However, the following may be indicators of pain:

- Facial changes, acute or chronic—for example, frozen watchfulness
- Sweating
- Increased heart rate and blood pressure
- Crying
- Reduced oxygenation of the blood, increased carbon dioxide
- Bronchospasm and increased pulmonary vascular resistance.

Keeping a diary

A diary (Appendix C) may prove valuable in helping parents and professionals to understand and manage chronic pain in children.

WAYS OF CHARTING PAIN

Charts for documenting pain scores can be used alongside those for recording other nursing observations such as pulse rate, temperature and blood pressure. We recommend that charts used in children's units are individually modified to include pain assessment measures for all postoperative patients. Completion of such charts (Appendix D) should prompt re-evaluation of analgesic efficacy, adverse effects (sedation, respiratory depression, cardiovascular changes, nausea and vomiting, etc.) and checks on infusion devices and delivery systems.[16] (The examples given are based on charts used at the Royal Hospital for Sick Children, Glasgow.)

The frequency with which pain scores should be recorded will vary with the nature of the problem. Titration of the use of analgesic drugs against their effectiveness should be an integral part of the assessment of pain control and this is facilitated by hourly assessments until the analgesia is stopped.

REFERENCES

1 Wong DL, Baker CM. Pain in children: comparison of assessment scales. *Pediatr Nursing* 1988;**14**:9–17.

2 Bellman MH, Paley CE. Pain control in children. Parents underestimate children's pain. *BMJ* 1993;**307**:1563.

3 Manne SL, Jacobsen PB, Redd WH. Assessment of acute pediatric pain: do child self report, parent rating and nurse ratings measure the same phenomena? *Pain* 1992;**48**:45–52.

4 Bieri D, Reeve RA, Champion GD, *et al.* The faces pain scale for the self-assessment of the severity of pain experienced by children: development, initial validation, and preliminary investigations for ratio scale properties. *Pain* 1990; **41**:139–50.

5 McGrath PA, Seifert CE, Speechley KN, *et al.* A new analogue scale for assessing children's pain: an initial validation study. *Pain* 1996;**64**:435–43.

6 Beyer JE, Wells N. The assessment of pain in children. *Pediatr Clin North Am* 1989;**36**:837–54.

7 Eland JM. Minimizing pain associated with pre-kindergarten intramuscular injections. *Iss Compr Pediatr Nurs* 1981;**5**:361–72.

8 Varni JW, Thompson KL, Hanson V. The Varni/Thompson pediatric pain questionnaire, 1 Chronic musculoskeletal pain in juvenile rheumatoid arthritis. *Pain* 1987;**28**:27–38.

9 Savedra MC, Tesler MD, Holzemerwl, Ward JA. *Adolescent pain tool: preliminary users manual.* San Francisco: University of California, 1989.

10 McGrath PA, de Veber LL, Hearn MJ. Multidimensional pain assessment in children. In: Fields HL, Dubner R, Cerveros R, eds. *Advances in pain and research therapy.* New York: Raven Press, 1985;**9**:387–93.

11 Katz ER, Kellerman J, Siegel SB. Behavioural distress in children with cancer undergoing medical procedures: Developmental considerations. *J Consult Clin Psychol* 1980;**48**:356–65.

12 Jay S, Olins M, Elliott CH, Caldwell S. Assessment of children's distress during painful medical procedures. *Hlth Psychol* 1983;**2**:133–47.

13 McGrath PJ, Johnson G, Goodman JT, *et al.* CHEOPS: a behavioural scale for rating post-operative pain in children. In: Fields HL, Dubner R, Cervero R, eds. *Advances in pain research and therapy.* New York: Raven Press, 1985;**9**: 395–402.

14 Gauvain-Piquard A, Rodary C, Rezvani A, Lemerle J. Pain in children aged 2–6 years: A new observational rating scale elaborated in a pediatric oncology unit—preliminary report. *Pain* 1987;**31**:177–88.

15 Beyer JE, McGrath PJ, Berde CB. Discordance between self-report and behavioural pain measures in children aged 3–7 years after surgery. *J Pain Symptom Man* 1990;**5**:350–6.

16 Morton NS. Development of a monitoring protocol for the safe use of opioids in children. *Paediatr Anaes* 1993;**3**:179–84.

14

3 Methods of pain relief

Note: Many of the following doses and/or preparations are not covered by a Product Licence or Summary of Product Characteristics. Their use is permitted by the Medicines Act, but practitioners must have adequate information to support their use.

The methods of pain relief discussed in this chapter are summarised in Box 3.1.

Box 3.1—Methods of pain relief

Systemically active drugs
- Non-opioid analgesics
  — paracetamol
  — non-steroidal anti-inflammatory drugs
  — salicylates
- Opioid analgesics
  Weak opioids
  Strong opioids
  — morphine
  — fentanyl
  — diamorphine
- Entonox

Local anaesthetics
- Lignocaine
- Bupivacaine
- Prilocaine
- EMLA and Ametop

Non-pharmacological interventions
- Environmental factors
- Supportive and distractive techniques
- Hypnosis
- Acupuncture
- Music and art therapy
- Desensitisation

Sedatives
- Chloral hydrate
- Midazolam
- Temazepam
- Ketamine

Pharmacological methods of pain relief include the use of both systemically active drugs and locally acting anaesthetic agents.

SYSTEMICALLY ACTIVE DRUGS

Most systemically active drugs used in pain control act on the central nervous system, but some, such as non-steroidal anti-inflammatory drugs (NSAIDs), act peripherally. The main distinction to be made is between non-opioid and opioid analgesics.

Non-opioid analgesics

The non-opioid analgesics (paracetamol, NSAIDs) have analgesic, antipyretic and anti-inflammatory properties in varying degrees. The analgesic most widely used in paediatric practice is probably paracetamol.

Box 3.2—Paracetamol formulations and dosage

Oral paracetamol
- Suspension: 120 mg/5 ml or 250 mg/5 ml (sugar free forms preferred; colorant free forms may be indicated for specific children; strawberry or banana flavours available)
- Tablets: 500 mg/soluble tablets: 500 mg
- Loading dose: 20 mg/kg
- Maintenance dose: 15 mg/kg
- Maximum daily dose: 90 mg/kg (60 mg/kg in neonates and infants)
- Dosing intervals: give no more often than every 4 h
- Do not give maximum daily dose for more than 72 h

or		
3–12 months	60–120 mg per dose
1–5 years	120–240 mg per dose
6–12 years	250–500 mg per dose

Rectal paracetamol[1]
- Suppositories: 60 mg, 125 mg, 250 mg, 500 mg, 1 g
- Loading dose: 30 mg/kg (20 mg/kg in neonates and infants)
- Maintenance dose: 20 mg/kg (15 mg/kg in neonates and infants)
- Maximum daily dose: 90 mg/kg/24 h (60 mg/kg in neonates and infants)
- Dosing intervals: give no more often than every 6 h
- Do not give maximum daily dose for more than 72 h

or		
Under 3 months	30–60 mg per dose
3–12 months	60–125 mg per dose
1–5 years	125–250 mg per dose
6–12 years	250–500 mg per dose

Paracetamol

Paracetamol is thought to work by inhibiting cyclo-oxygenase in the central nervous system but not in other tissues, so that it produces analgesia with no anti-inflammatory effect. It does not cause respiratory depression. It has a bad taste which has to be disguised.

The drug can be given orally or rectally (Box 3.2). Oral paracetamol is well absorbed from the upper small bowel (within 60 min) if gastric emptying is not delayed. Rectal paracetamol is poorly and slowly (90–120 min) absorbed and is thus a slow-release form of the drug, needing a larger loading dose and longer dosing interval.

Doses above those given in Box 3.2 do not give additional analgesia. Paracetamol is increasingly being used in combination with NSAIDs, weak opioids and strong opioids as part of a multimodal approach to the control of moderate or severe pain. Paracetamol can be very dangerous in overdose, and is contraindicated in children with severe liver disease.

Non-steroidal anti-inflammatory drugs (NSAIDs)
NSAIDs (Box 3.3) are powerful anti-inflammatory and antipyretic drugs with reasonably strong analgesic properties. They are

---

Box 3.3—NSAIDs: some formulations and dosages

Oral ibuprofen
- Suspension: 100 mg/5 ml, e.g. Brufen syrup (contains orange, sugar)
- Tablets: 200 mg, 400 mg, 600 mg
- Dose: 4–10 mg/kg every 6–8 h
- or   1–2 years   50 mg every 6–8 h
           3–7 years   100 mg every 6–8 h
           8–12 years   200 mg every 6–8 h

Oral diclofenac
- Tablets: enteric coated, 25 mg, 50 mg; soluble 50 mg (useful for smaller doses—dissolve in known quantity of water and take appropriate proportion)
- Dose: 0·5–1·5 mg/kg every 8–12 h
- Maximum daily dose: 3 mg/kg or 150 mg
- Oral diclofenac is not active until the enteric-coated tablets leave the stomach, that is more than 1 h after the dose. It is therefore unsuitable for acute pain relief or where there is delayed gastric emptying or poor gastrointestinal motility

Rectal diclofenac
- Suppositories: 12·5 mg, 25 mg, 50 mg, 100 mg
- Dose: 0·5–1·0 mg/kg every 8–12 h
- Maximum daily dose: 3 mg/kg
- Diclofenac is rapidly absorbed from the rectum (less than 60 min)

---

tolerated less well than paracetamol, with more chance of side effects. Children appear less prone than adults to the latter, but gastric irritation and platelet disorders are more likely after long term treatment.[2] Bronchospasm can be an acute complication, particularly in patients with unstable asthma. NSAIDs can be used in combination with paracetamol.

There are other NSAIDs, such as naproxen, which may be used. Ibuprofen has been shown to have the least risk of serious gastro-intestinal side effects (Committee on Safety of Medicines (CSM) 1996), and is therefore the preferred first choice. However, there is a variability in individual responses to different NSAIDs and some children may respond better to naproxen or diclofenac.

Only one NSAID should be used at a time. NSAIDs are particularly good for the control of:

- Mild to moderate musculoskeletal pain
- Inflammation of soft tissues and joints
- Pain from bony metastases
- Postoperative pain
- Pain after dental extraction
- Some colicky pains such as ureteric colic (unlike opioids, NSAIDs do not increase the contractility of visceral smooth muscle).

Used in combination with opioids, NSAIDs allow the use of a lower dose of opioid to achieve equivalent analgesia ("opioid-sparing effect"). They are also useful as a "step across" or "step down" analgesic when weaning a patient up or down the WHO ladder of pain control.

Cautions and contraindications NSAIDs are contraindicated if there is a history of or predisposition to gastrointestinal bleeding or ulceration. They should be avoided whenever possible if there is significant renal impairment. The drugs may interfere with platelet function and therefore should not be used in patients with thrombocytopenia or coagulation abnormalities, those receiving anticoagulant therapy or where there is a significant risk of postoperative bleeding.

NSAIDs should be used with caution in children with a tendency to asthma. Parents should be counselled to look for worsening symptoms, whereupon they should stop NSAID therapy immediately and seek medical advice. NSAIDs should be avoided in children receiving regular anti-asthma therapy (regular inhaled steroids/beta-agonists/oral steroids/inhaled cromoglycate).

NSAIDs are not licensed to be used in infants and should be used with care in this age group or in children weighing less than 10 kg.

Salicylates

Salicylates are powerful anti-inflammatory and antipyretic agents and reasonably strong analgesic drugs. However, they are gastric irritants and epidemiologically linked with Reye's syndrome. For the latter reason they are not licensed for use in children under 12 years, except in serious illnesses such as rheumatoid arthritis.

Opioid analgesics

The analgesia produced by opioid analgesics is specific and not part of the general brain depression that occurs with anaesthetic drugs. Most act on both the central and peripheral nervous systems. The side effects and problems associated with their use include respiratory depression and sedation. There may also be nausea and vomiting, constipation—as a result of decreased bowel peristalsis and increased sphincter muscle tone—and delayed gastric emptying, as well as urinary retention and pruritus. Tolerance may occur with opioid use. It is defined as a decreased effectiveness that develops after repeated administration of a drug, so that increasing doses are required to maintain clinical efficacy. Tolerance varies greatly between patients but may begin after 24 h in children. It appears more rapidly when opioids are given intravenously than when they are given by other routes.[3] Evidence from adult patients suggests that most patients with cancer do not require much dose escalation; usually most escalation is required because of progression of the disease.

Dependence is very rarely a problem when opioids are used for control of pain. Physical dependence occurs when repeated administration of a drug produces an altered physiological state; this state necessitates continued administration of the drug to prevent the appearance of a stereotypical withdrawal or absence syndrome characteristic of the drug. Gradual weaning from the drug is therefore required.

Psychological dependence on a drug (addiction) involves a behavioural pattern of drug use that is characterised by obsession with use of the drug (compulsive use) and securing its supply, and a strong tendency to relapse after withdrawal.

We shall consider separately the two classes of opioid analgesics: the weak opioids such as codeine, and the strong opioids such as morphine.

Weak opioids

Weak opioids have a "ceiling effect", that is their analgesic power does not increase beyond a certain dose. However, with increasing doses, side effects such as respiratory depression will occur. Codeine (Box 3.4) can be used alone or with paracetamol[4] or with NSAIDs.

Box 3.4—Codeine: a weak opioid

- Tablets: 15 mg, 30 mg
- Linctus: 15 mg/5 ml (sugar free); syrup 25 mg/5 ml
- Dose: 0·5–1 mg/kg every 4–6 h
- Good oral bioavailability

It is also an antitussive and antidiarrhoeal agent, and does not mask the neurological signs of head injury. Constipation is very likely with codeine use, so a laxative should be given prophylactically. Respiratory depression caused by codeine is reversed with naloxone.

Cautions Use codeine with caution in asthma and respiratory infection. The drug should never be given intravenously because of a high risk of causing hypotension and apnoea. Codeine should be used with caution in infants below 3 months of age. It should not be used in patients with renal impairment.

Dihydrocodeine may be prescribed by some paediatricians, but we have found little evidence to show that this drug is superior to codeine.

Strong opioids

When strong opioids are given for acute pain, professionals experienced in airway management and respiratory support must be immediately available at all times. Their use requires adequate monitoring of sedation level, respiratory function (that is, oxygen and carbon dioxide levels) and airway control. Strong opioids are contraindicated in the presence of airway obstruction, and should be used with caution in combination with any sedative, as the two drugs together may produce more respiratory depression than either given alone.

Strong opioids can be given by a variety of routes, each with benefits and drawbacks (Box 3.5). Particular care is required if an infusion device is used.

Safety of infusion devices All paediatric infusions should be regarded as high risk and an appropriate standard of infusion device

---

Box 3.5—Routes of administration of strong opioids: benefits and drawbacks

Oral
- Strong opioids are metabolised in the liver, reducing their bioavailability
- Peak effects are noticeable only after several doses

Rectal
- Rectal administration of opioids may reduce liver metabolism
- Useful if there is vomiting or ileus, but bioavailability is variable
- Older children in particular may dislike use of suppositories

Subcutaneous
- Subcutaneous delivery of opioids avoids liver metabolism, but drug levels are less predictable than with intravenous administration
- Infusion is through a small (24–25 g) cannula inserted after use of local anaesthetic cream
- Cannulae should be centrally placed (for example, in the abdominal wall, upper arms—deltoid region or thighs) to minimise the effect on absorption of variable peripheral perfusion. However, the child's preference for site is important
- For postoperative analgesia, insert a cannula during the operation
- Subcutaneous administration requires more concentrated solutions of morphine or diamorphine (see page 24)

continued

Box 3.5—*continued*

- Where peripheral perfusion is likely to be impaired, restoration of the circulation to the skin may cause a washout of the subcutaneous opioid depot[5]
- Unexpected reduction in effect could be due to precipitation in the tissues if high drug concentrations are used

Intramuscular
- An intramuscular cannula can be placed during anaesthesia or after use of local anaesthetic cream, and has the same advantages and limitations as a subcutaneous cannula
- When placed under anaesthesia, an intramuscular cannula can be used to provide short term emergence analgesia after operation

Intravenous
- Use a loading bolus dose and then continuous infusion
- Use preservative free morphine sulphate (causes less phlebitis)
- To manage acute pain:
  — use a dedicated cannula or antireflux valve
  — a bacterial filter may be used
  — use an anti-free flow (also called antisyphon) device to avoid inadvertent large doses

Spinal and epidural
- Spinal and epidural administration of strong opioids produces less intense analgesia than that achieved with local anaesthetics, without the latters' motor or sensory nerve side effects
- Analgesia from a single injection is prolonged, but with a high incidence of side effects (nausea and vomiting, urinary retention, itching and, rarely, hypotension and respiratory depression)
- Use preservative-free filtered solutions
- Can be used in combination with local anaesthetics (for example, diamorphine plus bupivacaine)
- Respiratory depression may occur up to 20 h after the last dose of opioid has been given
- If opioid extradural analgesia is to be used, a urinary catheter should be inserted at the time of operation—except in infants, whose bladder can often be expressed manually

must be used. Correct operation of the infusion device should be checked regularly and recorded along with residual volume in the infusion syringe. The infusion delivery system, from the pump to the patient, requires regular inspection to ensure its integrity and patency. The contents of each infusion syringe should be clearly recorded on the syringe and on a prescription chart, and before administration should be checked by a second professional and the chart countersigned with date and time (**see warning on page 7**).

Patient monitoring When a patient is receiving opioid drugs, the degree of monitoring required depends on whether the drugs are being used for acute or chronic pain. In palliative care, for example, where the priority is pain relief and the child's breathing is likely to become irregular as the disease progresses, it may be unhelpful to monitor respiratory function.

Hourly observations are usually appropriate for most children with acute pain. They should be more frequent, or even continuous, if the patient is unstable, pain control is poor or side effects are prominent. Children in neonatal or paediatric intensive care units need continuous observations. Major postoperative cases involving opioid analgesia need high dependency (1:2) or intensive (1:1) nursing care. When opioid infusions are used in a general ward, it is desirable to ensure that the minimum nurse to patient ratio is 1 nurse per 4 patients. These nurses should be appropriately trained in the care of sick children.

Parameters to monitor are:

- Pain relief: at rest and on movement
- Conscious level
- Oxygen saturation
- Respiratory rate
- Syringe movement
- Site of infusion
- Presence of nausea or vomiting
- Presence of constipation
- Presence of pruritus
- Presence of urinary retention.

Conscious level   The most sensitive indicator of significant opioid overdose is the conscious level or sedation score, particularly when these are charted serially. However, in a child receiving regular opioids for pain relief as part of palliative care, a fall in conscious level is most likely to be related to progression of the disease.

Oxygen saturation   Measurement of oxygen saturation (SaO_2) using a pulse oximeter is desirable. However, falling oxygen saturation can only act as an early warning sign of significant respiratory depression when room air is being breathed. When extra oxygen is being given, reduced oxygen saturation will be a late sign, occurring when arterial carbon dioxide tension is already high. Measurement of the partial pressure of carbon dioxide (ideally continuously using a transcutaneous monitor and backed up when appropriate by the measurement of arterial, capillary or central venous samples) can be useful in this situation. Children who are receiving opioids for the control of acute pain and needing additional inspired oxygen will require high dependency or intensive care. Lung volume may fall in the absence of a fall in oxygen saturation or an increase in arterial carbon dioxide tension.

Respiratory rate   As severe pain can increase respiratory rate, measurement of the latter can be a poor and late guide to opioid overdosage,[6] except in infancy where the presence of irregular breathing with apnoeic pauses of more than 12 s is a good indicator of overdose. However, a reduced respiratory rate should rouse suspicion of respiratory depression in children receiving opioids to control acute pain (Table 3.1).

Table 3.1 *Respiratory rates that may indicate respiratory depression in children receiving opioids for acute pain*

Age	Respiratory rate
Below 6 months	Below 20/min
6 months–2 years	Below 16/min
2–10 years	Below 14/min
Above 10 years	Below 12/min

Treatment with morphine

In children from 6 months to 5 years of age, morphine is metabolised more rapidly than in the adult, whereas in preterm and term neonates it is metabolised more slowly. The elimination half life of morphine is 6–20 h in neonates, 3–4 h in infants less than 6 months, less than 2 h in young preschool children, and 2 h in adults.

Oral morphine Morphine is extremely valuable orally, especially in chronic pain, being well absorbed from the gastrointestinal tract. Dosing is every 4 h or, with controlled-release preparations, every 8–12 h. Short-acting preparations include Oramorph liquid (10 mg, 30 mg, 100 mg/5 ml) and Sevredol tablets (10 mg, 20 mg, 50 mg); longer acting include MST Continus tablets (5 mg, 10 mg, 15 mg, 30 mg, 60 mg, 100 mg, 200 mg) and MST Continus suspension (20 mg, 30 mg, 60 mg, 100 mg, 200 mg/5 ml). The taste of oral morphine is usually acceptable.

For **acute pain control**, **oral** morphine starting doses are:

- Age 1–12 years: 200–400 microgram/kg every 4 h
- Age over 12 years: 10–15 mg every 4 h.

See pages 58–60 for use of morphine in neonates.

For **chronic pain control**, **oral** morphine starting doses are:

- Infants: 80–160 microgram/kg every 4 h
- For older children with chronic pain, starting doses of immediate release oral morphine are: 250–300 microgram/kg per dose every 4 hours giving a double dose at bedtime to avoid night-time waking
- For older children with chronic pain, starting doses of controlled release morphine are 750–1000 microgram/kg per dose every 12 hours or 500–650 microgram/kg per dose every 8 hours.

With continued treatment, tolerance may develop necessitating larger doses. The risk of morphine dependence is very low when the drug is used for pain control in children.

Rectal morphine Suppositories of 15 and 30 mg are available. The dose is the same as for oral morphine and their duration of action is 4 h.

Intravenous morphine may be given as a single dose, for example, before an invasive procedure, or as an infusion after a loading dose (see Tables 8.1 and 8.2 in Chapter 8). Preparations available for injection are 10 mg in 1 ml, and more concentrated solutions of 15 mg in 1 ml, 20 mg in 1 ml, 30 mg in 1 ml and 100 mg in 5 ml. **All commercially available preparations are extremely concentrated for infants and young children (see warning on page 7).** They can be diluted with 5%/10% dextrose or 0·9% saline. Typical loading doses are as follows:

- Infants: 100–150 microgram/kg over 30–60 min
- Age 1–12 years: 100–200 microgram/kg over 5–20 min
- Age over 12 years: 2·5–10·0 mg over 5–20 min.

Infusion is then at the rate of 10–50 microgram/kg/h (10–20 microgram/kg/h for neonates). Boluses may also be given (Table 3.2) **as an alternative to** an infusion.

When constituting morphine infusions for children under 50 kg in weight, a useful working concentration of morphine is: 1 mg/kg in 50 ml of 5% glucose or 0·9% saline to a maximum of 50 mg in 50 ml. Infusion of 1 ml/hour of this concentration = 20 microgram/kg per hour.

Table 3.2 *Intravenous morphine: bolus doses*

Age	Dose	Frequency
1–3 months	25 microgram/kg	Every 6 h
3–6 months	50 microgram/kg	Every 6 h
6–12 months	100 microgram/kg	Every 4–6 h
1–12 years	100–200 microgram/kg	Every 4–6 h
Over 12 years	2·5–10·0 mg	Every 4–6 h

These boluses are usually too large to be given in a patient already receiving an infusion of morphine.

Alternatives to morphine

Other strong opioids are fentanyl and diamorphine (see below and pages 58–9).

Fentanyl can be given orally, transdermally or intravenously.

Oral (transmucosal) fentanyl is given as fentanyl citrate in the form of a lollipop (15–20 microgram/kg) that is sucked by the child for 20–30 min. It has been found to be a safe and effective analgesic for bone marrow aspiration or lumbar puncture.[7] However, vomiting and itching occurred in a significant proportion of the patients in this trial, and further research is necessary to evaluate this approach.

Transdermal fentanyl The use of transdermal fentanyl is being researched.

Intravenous fentanyl is unsafe outside the intensive care unit or the operating theatre and must be supervised by an anaesthetist or intensivist. Fentanyl has fewer sedative/hypnotic properties than morphine, but it is a powerful respiratory depressant. Its action is of rapid onset (1 min) and brief duration (30–45 min). A loading dose of 1–5 microgram/kg is given slowly over 5 min to avoid causing chest wall rigidity. Subsequently a fentanyl infusion of 1–8 microgram/kg/h will usually require assisted ventilation. Fentanyl is useful during operations to augment inhaled anaesthetics.

Buprenorphine is available as sublingual tablets. However, in the event of an adverse reaction, reversal of the drug's effects is difficult and incomplete, and we do not advise the use of this drug for acute pain control in children. It may be useful for chronic pain control.

Patient controlled analgesia with morphine

Patient controlled analgesia[8,9] is suitable for any child able to understand the concept and physically operate the demand button on the pump that delivers the analgesic. Around 5 years is the youngest age at which patient controlled analgesia is usually applicable and effective.

The patient is first given a loading dose of 100–200 microgram/kg of morphine. Infusion of 1 ml/h of this concentration = 20 microgram/kg/h.

Always begin patient controlled analgesia with a background infusion of 2–8 microgram/kg/h of morphine (ideally 4 microgram/kg/h). A useful working concentration of morphine is: 1 mg/kg in 50 ml of 5% glucose or 0·9% saline to a maximum of 50 mg in 50 ml. A background infusion is particularly helpful in patients under 12 years of age and especially in the first 24–48 h of use when it can improve the child's sleeping pattern. Reduce and tail off the infusion as pain reduces and as adjuvant medication such as an NSAID is introduced and becomes effective.

Set the pump to deliver a suitable bolus dose. Boluses of 20 microgram/kg of morphine are usually appropriate. The maximum dose of morphine to be given in any 4 h period is 400 microgram/kg, and the optimum lockout interval (minimum time between doses) can vary from 5 to 15 min. It is better to reduce the lockout interval rather than increase the size of the bolus dose if analgesia is inadequate.

In older children (above 50 kg), use an adult pattern of patient controlled analgesia, that is, no background infusion, boluses of 1–2 mg with a 5–10 min lockout interval. The protocol for patient controlled analgesia must ensure that only the child—not the parents or nurses—can trigger the bolus doses.

Nurse controlled analgesia with morphine

Nurse controlled analgesia is of particular value in preschool children too young to manage patient controlled analgesia.

The child is first loaded with 100–200 microgram/kg of morphine. The background infusion of morphine is usually 10–20 microgram/kg/h. Boluses of morphine (10–20 microgram/kg) are given at the discretion of a single named nurse only, and not by the child or parents.

The lockout times vary from 30–60 min, and the maximum dose of morphine to be given in any 4 h period is 400 microgram/kg.

For maximum benefit from nurse controlled analgesia, painful procedures such as physiotherapy, turning, chest drain removal, should be anticipated and boluses given 5–10 min before each procedure.

Managing the side effects of powerful opioid drugs

Important side effects of strong opioids are listed in Box 3.6 and their management will be discussed in turn.

Box 3.6—Side effects of strong opioid drugs

- Respiratory depression
- Excessive sedation
- Nausea/vomiting
- Pruritus
- Constipation
- Urinary retention
- Muscle spasms

Respiratory depression

In the presence of respiratory depression, maintenance of airway, breathing and circulation is the priority, using basic and advanced paediatric life support measures.[10] If necessary give oxygen. Stop the infusion and check the pump, delivery system and contents of the infusion for integrity, patency and errors. If the infusion is correct and the child still needs the same degree of analgesia, and this cannot be given in any other form, then respiration should be supported artificially. (Use intubation and traditional positive pressure ventilation or, if available, non-invasive techniques. These include positive pressure ventilation by nasal mask or negative extrathoracic pressure ventilation by cuirass or tank respirator.)

If powerful analgesia is no longer needed, again apply basic and advanced life support techniques, and give naloxone 2–4 microgram/kg as an intravenous bolus repeated up to 10 microgram/kg. Naloxone's action is shorter than the respiratory depressant effects of morphine and therefore consider setting up an infusion of naloxone (10 microgram/kg/h) to maintain reversal.

Naloxone is available in two strengths, 20 microgram/ml and 400 microgram/ml. It can be given intramuscularly, subcutaneously or intraosseously if the intravenous route is not available.

Side effects of naloxone use include return of pain and nausea and vomiting.

Do not delay resuscitation while waiting for naloxone to take effect.

Naloxone reverses respiratory depression induced by all opioid drugs, including codeine.

Excessive sedation

If sedation is excessive, reduce or stop the opioid infusion, and if appropriate start resuscitation (airway, breathing, circulation).

Nausea/vomiting

Preparations available to control nausea and vomiting are listed in Box 3.7.

Cyclizine is an antihistamine which is valuable for both acute and chronic pain control. It is only weakly sedative and is particularly useful in treating opioid induced nausea associated with the control of long term pain and in terminal care.

Cyclizine can be given orally, rectally, by subcutaneous or intravenous infusion or by intravenous injection.

Side effects include slight sedation, dry mouth and occasionally blurred vision.

If the child is unresponsive to cyclizine, or a very emetic chemotherapy is being given, ondansetron may be effective.

Pruritus

Itching induced by opioids can be treated with the antihistamine chlorpheniramine at the following doses:

- Age under 1 year: 1 mg every 12 h (not recommended)
- Age 1–5 years: 1–2 mg every 8 h
- Age 6–12 years: 2–4 mg every 6–8 h
- Age over 12 years: 4 mg every 6–8 h.

Box 3.7—Drugs to control nausea and vomiting caused by opioids

Intravenous cyclizine
- 50 mg/ml
- Dose (every 8–12 h)
  - — Under 10 kg: 1 mg/kg
  - — 1–4 years (over 10 kg): 12·5 mg
  - — 5–12 years: 25 mg
  - — Over 12 years: 25–50 mg

Oral cyclizine
- Tablets: 50 mg
- Dose (2–3 times daily)
  - — Under 10 kg: 1 mg/kg
  - — 1–4 years (over 10 kg): 12·5 mg
  - — 5–12 years: 25 mg
  - — Over 12 years: 25–50 mg

Intravenous ondansetron
- Ampoules: 2 mg/ml
- Dose
  - — 100–200 microgram/kg to a maximum of 8 mg, given slowly over 2–5 min. This can be repeated once more within a period of 24 h if needed. Wait at least 8 h before second dose

Oral ondansetron
- Tablets: 4 mg, 8 mg
- Dose (every 8–12 h)
  - — Under 1 year: 1 mg
  - — 1–4 years: 2 mg
  - — Over 4 years: 4 mg

Another widely prescribed anti-emetic, prochlorperazine may also be effective

Oral prochlorperazine (not for children under 10 kg)
- Tablets: 5 mg. Syrup:1 mg/ml
- Dose (every 8–12 h)
  - — 1–4 years: 1·25–2·5 mg
  - — 5–12 years: 2·5–5·0 mg
  - — Over 12 years: 5·0–10·0 mg
- Prochlorperazine should not be given intravenously
- Small risk of extrapyramidal side effects

Rectal prochlorperazine
- Suppositories: 5 mg, 25 mg
- Dose: 150–250 microgram/kg
- Maximum frequency: every 8 h

Intramuscular prochlorperazine
- Ampoules: 12·5 mg/ml
- Dose: 150–250 microgram/kg
- Maximum frequency: every 8 h

For the pruritus induced by spinal or epidural opioids, naloxone in smaller doses than that given for respiratory depression is effective without reversing the analgesia.[11] Give a loading dose of 0·5 microgram/kg repeated at 10–15 min intervals as necessary up to a total of 2 microgram/kg then infuse at 1–2 microgram/kg/h. Naloxone has the advantage of not potentiating sedation as can occur with alternatives such as antihistamines.

Constipation

The pain of constipation resulting from opioid drugs can be severe and should be prevented. Combinations of bulk forming, stimulant osmotic laxatives and faecal softening drugs should be used prophylactically to prevent constipation or treat constipation if it becomes established.

Occasionally, suppositories such as bisacodyl and micro-enemas may be required.

Urinary retention

Urinary retention can usually await a fall in opioid levels but if analgesia needs to be maintained at the same level, a catheter may be required. When retention results from epidural opioid treatment, a small dose of naloxone as indicated for pruritus can be of value.

Muscle spasms

Muscle spasms may occur after orthopaedic procedures in children receiving opioid infusions. Use a morphine sparing co-analgesic, for example, ibuprofen (4–10 mg/kg, every 6–8 h) and consider oral diazepam (100 microgram/kg every 6 h).

Prescription of controlled drugs

Requirements for the prescription of controlled drugs in the UK are set out in the *British National Formulary.*

Prescriptions ordering controlled drugs must be signed and dated by the prescriber and specify the prescriber's address. The prescription must always state in the prescriber's own handwriting, in ink or otherwise so as to be indelible, the following:

- The name and address of the patient
- In the case of a preparation, the form and where appropriate the strength of the preparation
- The total quantity of the preparation, or the number of dose units, in both words and figures
- The dose.

A prescription may order a controlled drug to be dispensed by instalments; the amount of the instalments and the intervals to be observed must be specified. Prescriptions ordering "repeats" on the same form are not permitted.

It is an offence for a doctor to issue an incomplete prescription and a pharmacist is not allowed to dispense a controlled drug unless all the information required by law is given on the prescription. Failure to comply with the regulations concerning the writing of prescriptions will cause inconvenience to patients and delay in supplying the necessary medicine.

The administration of sedative and analgesic drugs to children

In preparing a single dose or infusion, it is essential that two qualified members of the nursing and/or medical staff check the prescription, dose, formulation, dilution and administration to the patient of all drugs and in particular opioids. All parenterally given agents should be regarded as high risk since errors may produce immediate adverse or even fatal effects.

This is particularly important, when, for example, morphine is being administered to an infant or young child. The original ampoule of morphine usually contains 10 mg in 1 ml (that is 10,000 microgram in 1 ml). Dilution of this powerful solution can be potentially dangerous if great care is not taken. We recommend that hospital pharmacies prepare or obtain specially made up solutions of morphine for use in infants and young children (perhaps 1 mg in 1 ml).

Entonox

Nitrous oxide gas (Entonox) can be used to provide an inhalational form of patient controlled analgesia and the mask or mouthpiece should only be held by the patient, not the parent or nurse.[12]

Entonox is a colourless, odourless gas that will provide analgesia, with only weak anaesthesia, at a concentration of 50% nitrous oxide and 50% oxygen. The delivery apparatus is most often used on a demand basis, that is, the drug is delivered when the patient inhales, and Entonox analgesia is a valuable supportive therapy in acute trauma and procedural pain.

A mask or mouthpiece can be used to deliver Entonox, and portable, lightweight equipment is available with clear shell, soft rimmed masks and disposable mouthpieces. The child has to be cooperative to be able to inhale the gas, and using Entonox can be difficult in children under 7 years of age. This is clearly a safeguard, but weakens its effectiveness in distressed children.

Entonox takes 3–5 min to achieve peak effect, and then wears off over several minutes, making it ideal for outpatient procedures. Most experience with Entonox in children has been gained during dressing changes, particularly in patients with burns. It is also useful in the ambulance during transit to hospital.

Fasting before Entonox administration is usually unnecessary if it is used as the sole analgesic. Where other analgesics, opioids or sedatives are given, the child should be fasted as for a general anaesthetic, that is, no solids or milk for 6 h, no clear fluids for 3 h.

Entonox can also be used as a continuous inhalation at a rate of 6 l/min and diluted with air. As it does not usually produce complete loss of consciousness, it is important to talk with the child throughout administration. Entonox may infrequently cause vomiting and euphoria.

Cautions and contraindications Entonox should not be used after injuries to the head or chest that contain air, because diffusion of the gas into a closed space can increase pressure.[13] Entonox is also contraindicated in bowel obstruction. Caution is required when other sedatives or opioids have been or are being given, because sedation and respiratory depression will be potentiated. Entonox should not be used for prolonged periods as it may interfere with Vitamin B_{12} metabolism.

LOCAL ANAESTHETICS

Local anaesthetics can be injected centrally (around the spinal cord), regionally (around major nerve roots) or peripherally (around nerve endings). They reversibly block nerve conduction. Their duration of action depends on individual drug chemistry, on their local concentration and on whether or not they are used with a vasoconstrictor.

Systemic toxicity can occur as a result of excessive dosage, inadvertent intravenous injection or absorption through inflamed tissues. It can involve the central nervous system, where there is initial depression of inhibiting neurones and later excitation that can provoke convulsions.

Early signs of toxicity include circumoral numbness or tingling, muscle twitches, dizziness, tinnitus, light-headedness, slurred speech and aggression. Later and dangerous signs include fits, coma, respiratory arrest and cardiac arrhythmias, although with bupivacaine myocardial toxicity can occur early.

The maximum permissible dose of local anaesthetic depends upon the route of administration and the use of vasoconstrictors. Prevention of side effects and toxicity requires the avoidance of intravenous injection by frequent aspiration of the syringe. The use of a vasoconstrictor can reduce toxicity from a local anaesthetic, as well as extending the duration of action.

31

There should be immediate access to resuscitation equipment wherever local anaesthetics are in use. In the event of toxicity the drug should be stopped immediately and basic and advanced paediatric life support techniques started as required.[10]

Local anaesthetic drugs

Commonly used local anaesthetic drugs are lignocaine, bupivacaine and prilocaine.

Lignocaine

Lignocaine is a medium-acting agent, its effect lasting 30 min–2 h.

When used with adrenaline (1 in 200,000) the drug lasts for 2–4 h.

The maximum total dose of lignocaine given in any 4 h period is 4 mg/kg, whether it is used plain (without adrenaline) or with adrenaline. The total dose of adrenaline used should not exceed 7 microgram/kg, that is, 1·4 ml/kg of 1:200,000 solution.

Bupivacaine

Bupivacaine has a slower onset than lignocaine but is longer acting (3–7 h). It is more toxic to the heart. The maximum dose is 2·5 mg/kg in any 6 h period and by epidural top-up or infusion is 2 mg/kg in any 4 h period (1 mg/kg in neonates). There are only limited data on repeated dosing or infusion by other routes.

Prilocaine

Prilocaine is shorter acting than either lignocaine or bupivacaine. It is the least toxic of local anaesthetics except in neonates, in whom excess dosage may induce methaemoglobinaemia.

Prilocaine is usually applied as part of a eutectic mixture of local anaesthetics (2·5% prilocaine plus 2·5% lignocaine) formulated as EMLA cream. Prilocaine is the drug of choice for intravenous regional anaesthesia in older children (Bier's blocks).

Box 3.8

Concentrations of local anaesthetic drugs
- 2% = 20 mg/ml
- 1% = 10 mg/ml
- 0·5% = 5 mg/ml
- 0·25% = 2·5 mg/ml

Concentrations of adrenaline
- 1:1000 = 1000 microgram/ml
- 1:10,000 = 100 microgram/ml
- 1:100,000 = 10 microgram/ml
- 1:200,000 = 5 microgram/ml
- 1:400,000 = 2·5 microgram/ml

Methods of using local anaesthetics

Local anaesthetics can be applied topically as gels, creams or drops, infiltrated or infused, or injected to achieve nerve block.

Gels and creams

Local anaesthetic gels and creams are usually applied to the skin and covered by an occlusive pad to promote absorption. In toddlers, cover occlusive pads with bandages because the gel can be toxic if swallowed. Use the gels only on intact skin and not on mucosa or burned or inflamed skin. The gels can cause sensitisation on repeated exposure, so staff must take care when applying or removing them.

Eutectic mixture of local anaesthetics (EMLA)[14-16] consists of lignocaine 2·5% plus prilocaine 2·5%. It cannot be applied to open wounds or burns, and must not be used on mucous membranes or the anus. It has no product licence for use at under 1 year of age.

Squeeze one quarter to one half the contents of a 5 g tube on to the area to be treated, spread thickly and cover with the patch provided. Write the time of application on the patch. EMLA cream needs at least 45 min (ideally 60–90 min) to work; onset is slower in non-caucasians, because its absorption is impeded by melanin in the skin. It constricts capillaries in the skin, causing blanching. This constriction resolves 15 min after removal of the cream, although the analgesia persists for 1 h. Skin irritation may occur if the gel is left on for more than 2 h.

Amethocaine gel (Ametop)[17-19] contains 40 mg/g of amethocaine. It is not yet recommended for preterm babies or infants under 1 month of age.

Ametop is used in the same way as EMLA but, unlike EMLA, may dilate capillaries making the siting of cannulae easier. There is adequate analgesia after 30 min for venepuncture and after 45 min for venous cannulation. After removal of the gel (no longer than 1 h after application), anaesthesia remains for 4–6 h. Slight erythema, itching and oedema may occur at the site. The gel is available "over the counter" and is not a prescription only medicine. It can therefore be applied by parents before bringing their child to the hospital as a day case for venepunctures or other procedures.

Of course, this should not stop paediatricians prescribing it or EMLA so that parents can apply these preparations in advance of basic procedures.

Lignocaine 1% or 2% is available as a sterile lubricant loaded in a syringe and in tubes for installation into the urethra prior to urinary catheterisation. The usual dose is 3 mg/kg. The maximum dose is 4 mg/kg.

This anaesthetic gel can also be used at the site of a circumcision, either as the sole analgesic or to provide topical analgesia once the caudal or penile block is starting to wear off. Repeated application for up to 24 h and the avoidance of troublesome and ineffective dressings after circumcision help to keep patients comfortable.

Eye drops

Amethocaine or oxybuprocaine eye drops can be used to provide analgesia during eye surgery in children.

Infiltration and infusion

Lignocaine and bupivacaine can both be infiltrated around wounds to provide local analgesia.

For infiltration, 1% lignocaine is usually used, providing a rapid and intense block that is effective for up to 2 h. The usual dose is 3 mg/kg (to a maximum in the older child of 200 mg). Use fine needles (27–29 gauge) in the awake patient. Warming the solution to body temperature and injecting it very slowly can reduce the local stinging. Aspiration before each injection and constant movement of the needle are useful ways of minimising intravascular injections.

Lignocaine has a pH of 5 to improve its shelf life, and for this reason can be painful when injected. Use of a solution buffered with bicarbonate will lessen the pain associated with infiltration,[19] but local adrenaline cannot then be used as it is inactivated by the bicarbonate buffer. Buffered lignocaine comprises 1 part of 8·4% sodium bicarbonate to 10 parts of 1% lignocaine. This latter mixture maintains its pharmacological activity for 1 week at room temperature and for 2 weeks if kept in a refrigerator, but if made up on the ward should be used according to local policy within 24 h to limit possible microbial contamination.

Plain bupivacaine 0·25% is useful for infiltrating wound edges during surgery to provide postoperative pain relief. The analgesia is effective for up to 8 h and therefore particularly useful for day case surgery.

Local anaesthetics with vasoconstrictors can also be instilled into open wounds in the awake child before infiltration with a needle.[20] Wait for 2–5 min after instilling, and then infiltrate from inside to out via the anaesthetised area.

After thoracotomy, infiltration of the rib cage with 0·25% bupivacaine can provide effective postoperative pain control for around 12 h (maximum dose 2·5 mg/kg in any 6 h period).

Bupivacaine 0·25% can also be instilled onto dressings, for example those used for skin graft donor sites. Wounds can also be perfused by placing an epidural catheter into the wound before closure, then infusing 0·25% bupivacaine at 1–3 ml/h (maximum dose 2·5 mg/kg in any 6 h period).

Nerve blocks

Nerve blocks should be used only by those trained and experienced in providing regional anaesthesia. Usually the drug used is bupivacaine (0·25%) with a maximum dose of 2 mg/kg in a 4 h period. Vascoconstrictors must never be used with digital or penile nerve blocks.

Commonly used nerve blocks are:

- Digital nerve block for removal of fingernails or toenails (not with vasoconstrictors)
- Ilio-inguinal block for hernia repair
- Dorsal nerve of penis block for circumcision (not with vasoconstrictors)
- Axillary nerve block[21]
- Femoral nerve block (for example, for fractured femur) (see page 47).

Vasoconstrictors extend the duration of analgesia for a given dose of anaesthetic, but must not be used where arterial spasm may produce tissue damage, for example, with nerve blocks in the fingers, toes or penis.

When using a nerve block, ensure compartment syndrome is not present or developing and masked by the local analgesia. If a limb is encased in a cast, the circulation in the exposed fingers or toes should be checked regularly. If there is breakthrough pain, investigate to ensure the adequacy of circulation before giving further analgesia.

Intravenous block

Intravenous nerve block must be used only by a suitably trained and experienced anaesthetist, with full resuscitation facilities available. The technique is normally used to provide short-lasting anaesthesia of a limb—usually an arm to treat a fracture. Use prilocaine (not bupivacaine) as 0·5% solution, in a total dose of up to 4 mg/kg. Ensure that a double cuff, pneumatic tourniquet is used with close pressure monitoring.

Central (spinal cord) blocks

Central nerve blocks should be undertaken and supervised by a suitably trained and experienced anaesthetist. They can be given epidurally, with or without a catheter, in the caudal, lumbar or thoracic regions, or into the subarachnoid space (usually L3/L4 or L4/L5). Additives, such as preservative free clonidine[22,23] or preservative free ketamine[24] can be added to bupivacaine 0·25%. These may considerably prolong the duration of caudal blocks. Adrenaline should be avoided in epidural blocks undertaken in children.[25] Infants and children are less likely to show the hypotension that adults develop with spinal cord blocks. The numbness induced makes the patient vulnerable to pressure ischaemia, and may make it difficult to recognise swelling under a plaster cast. It is therefore important to watch for colour changes in the fingers or toes. Sheepskins can be helpful in protecting the skin from pressure ischaemia.

Epidural blocks may provoke short term urinary retention; this may require catheterisation unless the patient is young enough to have their bladder emptied by gentle suprapubic pressure.

Contraindications to the use of spinal cord blocks include local sepsis and coagulopathies.

NON-PHARMACOLOGICAL INTERVENTIONS

Environmental factors

An accident and emergency department or the treatment room on a paediatric ward can often be a frightening place for a child. Every attempt should be made to minimise or remove the negative aspects of these areas, such as an overly "clinical" appearance and evidence of invasive instrumentation, and create instead an attractive, decorated environment with toys, mobiles and pictures. Areas allowing privacy are essential.

Supportive and distractive techniques

We discuss here ways to support and distract children experiencing acute pain.[26–28] More long term strategies appropriate to the control of chronic pain are described in Chapter 9.

It is becoming more common for parents to stay with their child during an invasive procedure. However, this depends on the experience of the doctor and the type of procedure. Less experienced doctors are more uncomfortable with parents present, and many doctors will allow parents to stay for venepuncture or lumbar puncture but would exclude them during, for example, insertion of a chest drain.

In one study almost all children between the ages of 9 and 12 years reported that the "thing that helped most" was to have their parents present during a painful procedure.[29,30] It is not enough, however, just to allow parents to be present; they need guidance on how to support their child during the procedure. Studies suggest, for example, that talking to and touching a child during a procedure is both soothing and anxiety relieving. We recommend that parents are present with their child during invasive procedures, unless there are good medical reasons to exclude them.

The child and parents should be adequately prepared for the procedure. Explaining to the parents and child why the procedure is needed, how it will be done and how long it will take may help reduce anxiety.

Avoid use of the word "good" as in "good boy" or "good girl". A child may feel that if he or she cries or shouts this will be seen as naughty, whereas shouting may be an effective distraction strategy: "I don't mind you shouting, as long as you keep still".

Age appropriate distraction strategies include:

- Holding a familiar object (comforter), such as a pillow or soft cuddly toy
- Singing; concentrating on nice things; telling jokes; games and puzzles
- Going on imaginary journeys
- Blowing out air or bubbles[31]
- Reading pop-up books[32]
- Playing with a kaleidoscope or 3D viewer
- Breathing out (but not hyperventilation, which may increase anxiety and induce venoconstriction)
- Looking in a mirror to see the view through a nearby window
- Watching television or a video; playing interactive computer games
- Listening through headphones to stories or music.

Parents can assist with many of these activities. Another option is relaxation exercises, in which muscles are tensed in sequence and then relaxed.

Not all children are helped by distraction; some prefer to focus on the procedure. What is important is to identify each child's coping mechanism and help the child to use it. It is counter-productive if we attempt to impose our views (for example, that distraction is a good idea) on a child who does not wish to be distracted.

Hypnosis

Hypnosis is an altered state of consciousness, in which a child may perceive pain as less severe. It can be induced by helping the child to focus attention on a more pleasant alternative. There has been considerable work on the use of hypnosis in acute or procedural pain in children,[33-38] but few clinicians are familiar with the techniques, which are rarely used in clinical practice. According to hypnotic theory, however, hypnosis should be relatively simple to apply in an emergency situation, because the child is already in an "altered state of consciousness" brought about by an unfamiliar and potentially frightening environment. It is difficult, if not impossible, to use hypnosis in children with learning difficulties.

Only one of the authors of this manual has personal experience of hypnotherapy in pain relief. Sources of advice for interested practitioners are listed in Resources (see page 93).

Acupuncture

Acupuncture, part of traditional Chinese medicine, is reported to be effective treatment for some types of pain in adults, but few randomised controlled clinical studies have been carried out in children. Acupuncture could be a valuable and valid form of treatment in children, even though they tend to be afraid of needles but more research into its clinical effectiveness is required before it can be recommended.

Music and art therapy

These techniques may also be of value.[16]

Desensitisation

This may be necessary in a few children who require repeated procedures. A child psychologist, experienced in the technique, should be enlisted.

SEDATIVES AS ADJUVANTS TO ANALGESIA

As well as the supportive and distractive techniques described, psychotropic drugs may also be used to enhance pharmacological analgesia in children. Sedatives are particularly valuable when lengthy or repeated procedures are undertaken. However, sedatives may result in unpredictable responses in some children who may become disinhibited, agitated, restless or over-sedated and anaesthetised (that is, verbal contact is lost and protective airway reflexes are depressed or lost). Some sedative agents produce very prolonged sedation, and recovery to a suitable level to allow discharge home may be delayed. During their administration appropriate monitoring should be undertaken and skilled individuals should be available to manage the airway if a problem develops. Sedatives are contraindicated in infants or children with upper airway obstruction.

Sedatives relieve anxiety, not pain. They may reduce a child's ability to communicate discomfort and therefore should not be given in isolation. Remember that it may be difficult to sedate a child who is receiving anticonvulsants using normal doses of sedatives. Sedatives used in this setting include chloral hydrate, midazolam and temazepam. The anaesthetic ketamine may be used for short procedures.

Chloral hydrate

Chloral hydrate is a pure sedative/hypnotic with no analgesic properties. It should not be used alone for painful procedures. The solutions (200 mg/5 ml and 500 mg/5 ml) can be given orally with water or fruit juice or rectally, in doses of 25–50 mg/kg. Doses of 100 mg/kg can be given for procedures such as scanning or echocardiography where it is important for the child to lie still. The time to sedation is about 40 min and the recovery time about 60 min, although residual effects can persist for up to 24 h after administration.[39]

Unwanted side effects

Chloral hydrate may produce an agitated response, and it may cause gastric irritation. It may cause hypotension if combined with frusemide.

In young children with obstructed airways, chloral hydrate may cause worsening of upper airway obstruction during sleep.[40]

Midazolam

Midazolam is an amnesic sedative but not analgesic drug. It should not be used alone for painful procedures. The intravenous dose for procedures is 100–200 microgram/kg. The drug has a rapid action and is rapidly metabolised.

Midazolam is available for injection as 2 mg/ml and 5 mg/ml.

Midazolam can also be given orally[41,42] and intranasally[43,44] using the injection solution at a dose of 400–500 microgram/kg; onset is after 15 min and recovery after 1 h. The maximum dose is 15 mg, and in heavier children temazepam may be a good alternative. Midazolam solution is acidic (pH 3·3) and its taste should be disguised by formulating a syrup (2·5 mg/ml) (not yet commercially available) or by adding the dose to a small volume (1–2 ml/kg) of fruit juice, fizzy cola or lemonade.

In some children, midazolam causes respiratory depression and hyperexcitability. These can be reversed by flumazenil 10 microgram/kg. If this does not work, a further dose of 10 microgram/kg can be given, followed by an infusion of 10 microgram/kg/h.

When using midazolam, professionals experienced in airway management and respiratory support must be immediately available

39

at all times. Adequate respiratory and airway monitoring must be undertaken.

Temazepam

Temazepam is an alternative to midazolam for children weighing more than 30 kg. The drug is available in 10 mg and 20 mg capsules. The dose is 0·5–1·0 mg/kg, to a maximum of 20 mg.

Ketamine

Ketamine may produce laryngospasm, particularly in infants. It should therefore be given only by a trained anaesthetist or intensivist able to deal safely with acute upper airway obstruction. Fasting, as before general anaesthesia, is necessary before it is used (see page 4).

Ketamine is a potent analgesic as well as a dissociative anaesthetic. It can be used as an analgesic at doses much lower than those producing general anaesthesia. The dose for procedures is 1–4 mg/kg intravenously over a minimum of 60 s, to produce 5–10 min of surgical anaesthesia. Onset is rapid (1 min) as is recovery (15–20 min). For maintenance, an intravenous infusion of 10–45 microgram/kg/min can be given according to the response. Ketamine can also be given orally as a premedication for invasive procedures in a dose of between 2 and 10 mg/kg.[45]

Ketamine is available for injection as 10 mg/ml, 50 mg/ml and 100 mg/ml. The solution for injection can also be given orally.

Ketamine causes no significant hypotension and airway control is usually maintained; however in one study, one in 180 children had laryngospasm.[46,47] Respiratory arrest may also occur.[48] Many children, particularly infants, show increased airway secretions that may contribute to laryngospasm. Premedication with oral atropine (40 microgram/kg) or systemic atropine (20 microgram/kg) or glycopyrrolate (10 microgram/kg) may reduce secretions.

Ketamine should not be used after a head injury or in states of impaired consciousness. It is contraindicated in systemic hypertension and in intracranial problems. It can be used, but with caution, in children with pulmonary hypertension.[49] It may also be used in a much reduced dose in neonates; in the latter it can be a valuable drug for providing analgesia and dissociative anaesthesia for laser and cryotherapy for retinopathy.[50,51] This technique should only be undertaken by an experienced paediatric anaesthetist.

Ketamine can produce nightmares and hallucinations, especially in older children; for this reason premedication with a small dose of oral midazolam (maximum 250 microgram/kg) or intravenous midazolam 50 microgram/kg is appropriate. Adequate respiratory and airway monitoring must always be undertaken.

REFERENCES

1 Gaudreault P, Guay J, Nicol O, Dupuis C. Pharmacokinetics and clinical efficacy of intrarectal solution of acetaminophen. *Can J Anaesth* 1988;**35**: 149–52.
2 Shannon M, Berde CB. Pharmacologic management of pain in children and adolescents. *Pediatr Clinics North Am* 1989;**36(4)**:855–71.
3 Hanks GW, Twycross RG. Pain, the physiological antagonist of opioid analgesics. *Lancet* 1984;**1**:1477–8.
4 Tobias JD, Lowe S, Hersey S, Rasmussen GE, Werkhaven J. Analgesia after bilateral myringotomy and placement of pressure equalization tubes in children: acetaminophen versus acetaminophen with codeine. *Anesth Analg* 1995;**81**: 496–500.
5 Wolf AR, Lawson RA, Fisher S. Ventilatory arrest after a fluid challenge in a neonate receiving sc morphine. *Br J Anaesth* 1995;**75**:787–9.
6 Gerber N, Apseloff G. Death from a morphine infusion during a sickle cell crisis. *J Pediatr* 1993;**123**:322–5.
7 Schechter NL, Weisman SJ, Rosenblum M, Bernstein B, Conard PL. The use of oral transmucosal fentanyl citrate for painful procedures in children. *Pediatrics* 1995;**95**:335–9.
8 Doyle E, Harper I, Morton NS. Patient controlled analgesia with low dose background infusions after lower abdominal surgery in children. *Br J Anaesth* 1993;**71**:818–22.
9 Gillespie JA, Morton NS. Patient controlled analgesia for children: a review. *Paediatr Anaesth* 1992;**2**:51–9.
10 Mackway-Jones K, Phillips B, Molyneux E, Wieteska S, eds. *Advanced paediatric life support: the practical approach*, 2nd edn. London: BMJ Books, 1996.
11 Rose JB, Francis MC, Kettrick RG. Continuous naloxone infusion in paediatric patients with pruritis associated with epidural morphine. *Paediatr Anaesth* 1993; **3**:255–8.
12 Gamis AS, Knapp JF, Glenski JA. Nitrous oxide analgesia in a paediatric emergency department. *Ann Emerg Med* 1989;**18**:177–81.
13 Macrae WA, Davies HT. Pain from acute trauma. *Prescribers J* 1993;**33**:232–7.
14 Uhari M. A Eutectic mixture of lidocaine and prilocaine for alleviating vaccination pain in infants. *Pediatrics* 1993;**92**:719–21.
15 Maunuksela EL, Korpela R. Double blind valuation of a lignocaine–prilocaine cream (EMLA) in children. *Br J Anaesth* 1986;**58**:1242–5.
16 Arts SE, Abu-Saad HH, Champion GD, *et al.* Age-related response to lidocaine–prilocaine (EMLA) emulsion and effect of music distraction on the pain of intravenous cannulation. *Pediatrics* 1994;**93**:797–801.
17 Woolfson AD, McCafferty DF, Boston V. Clinical experiences with a novel percutaneous amethocaine preparation: prevention of pain due to venepuncture in children. *Br J Clin Pharmacol* 1990;**30**:273–9.
18 Lawson RA, Smart NG, Gudgeon AC, Morton NS. Evaluation of an amethocaine gel preparation for percutaneous analgesia before venous cannulation in children. *Br J Anaesth* 1995;**75**:282–5.
19 Klein EJ, Shugerman RP, Leigh-Taylor K, Schneider C, Portscheller D, Koepsell T. Buffered lidocaine: analgesia for intravenous line placement in children. *Pediatrics* 1995;**95**:709–12.
20 Smith GA, Stratusbaugh SD, Harbeck-Weber C, *et al.* Comparison of topical anesthetics without cocaine to tetracaine-adrenaline-cocaine and lidocaine infiltration during repair of lacerations: bupivacaine-norepinephrine is an effective new topical anesthetic agent. *Pediatrics* 1996;**97**:301–7.
21 Fewtrell MS, Sapsford DJ, Herrick MJ, Noble-Jamieson G, Ross Russell RI. Continuous axillary nerve block for chronic pain. *Arch Dis Child* 1994;**70**:54–5.
22 Lee JJ, Rubin AP. Comparison of a bupivacaine-clonidine mixture with plain bupivacaine for caudal analgesia in children. *Br J Anaesth* 1994;**72**:258–62.
23 Jamali S, Monin S, Begon C, Dubousset AM, Ecoffey C. Clonidine in pediatric caudal anesthesia. *Anesth Analg* 1994;**78**:663–6.
24 Cook B, Grubb DJ, Aldridge LA, Doyle E. Comparison of the effects of adrenaline, clonidine and ketamine on the duration of caudal analgesia produced by bupivacaine in children. *Br J Anaesth* 1995;**75**:698–701.

25 Goldman LJ. Complications in regional anaesthesia. *Paediatr Anaesth* 1995;**5**: 3–9.
26 Kuttner L. Management of young children's acute pain and anxiety during invasive medical procedures. *Paediatrician* 1989;**16**:39–44.
27 Kuttner L, Bowman M, Teasdale M. Psychological treatment of distress, pain and anxiety for young children with cancer. *J Dev Behav Pediatr* 1988;**9**:374–81.
28 Collier J, MacKinlay D, Watson AR. Painful procedures: preparation and coping strategies for children. *Mat Child Health* 1993;**18**:282–6.
29 Bauchner H, Waring C, Vinci R. Parental presence during procedures in an emergency room: results from fifty observations. *Pediatrics* 1991;**87**:544–8.
30 Bauchner H, Vinci R, Bak S, *et al.* Parents and procedures: a randomised controlled trial. *Pediatrics* 1996;**98**:861–7.
31 French GM, Painter EC, Coury DL. Blowing away shot pain: a technique for pain management during immunization. *Pediatrics* 1994;**93**:384–8.
32 Rogers F, Sharapan H, Lucchino J. *Tricks and more tricks*. USA: Family Communications, 1993.
33 Olness K. Hypnosis in paediatric practice. *Curr Prob Paediatr* 1981;**12**:1–47.
34 Olness K, Gardner GG. Some guidelines for uses of hypnotherapy in pediatrics. *Pediatrics* 1978;**62**:228–33.
35 Olness K, MacDonald J. Self hypnosis and biofeedback in the management of juvenile migraine. *J Dev Behav Pediatr* 1981;**2**:168–70.
36 Olness K, Wain HJ, Ng L. A pilot study of blood endorphin levels in children using self-hypnosis to control pain. *J Dev Behav Pediatr* 1980;**1**:187–8.
37 Kuttner L. Favorite stories: a hypnotic pain-reduction technique for children in acute pain. *Am J Clin Hyp* 1988;**30**:289–95.
38 Bernstein NR. Management of burned children with the aid of hypnosis. *J Child Psychol Psychiatr* 1963;**4**:93–8.
39 Cray SH, Hinton W. Sedation for investigations: prolonged effect of chloral and trimeprazine. *Arch Dis Child* 1994;**71**:179.
40 Biban P, Baraldi E, Pettenazzo A, Filippone M, Zacchello F. Adverse effect of chloral hydrate in two young children with obstructive sleep apnea. *Pediatrics* 1993;**92**:461–3.
41 Hennes HM, Wagner V, Bonadio WA, *et al.* The effect of oral midazolam on anxiety of preschool children during laceration repair. *Ann Emerg Med* 1990; **19**:1006–9.
42 Connors K, Terndrup TE. Nasal versus oral midazolam for sedation of anxious children undergoing laceration repair. *Ann Emerg Med* 1994;**24**:1074–9.
43 Yealy DM, Ellis JH, Hobbs GD, Moscati RM. Intranasal midazolam as a sedative for children during laceration repair. *Am J Emerg Med* 1992;**10**:584–7.
44 Theroux MC, West DW, Corddry DH, *et al.* Efficacy of intranasal midazolam in facilitating suturing of lacerations in preschool children in the emergency department. *Pediatrics* 1993;**91**:624–7.
45 Tobias JD Phipps S, Smith B, Mulhern RK. Oral ketamine premedication to alleviate the distress of invasive procedures in pediatric oncology patients. *Pediatrics* 1992;**90**:537–41.
46 Green SM, Johnson NE. Ketamine sedation for paediatric procedures: part two, review and implications. *Ann Emerg Med* 1990;**19**:1033–46.
47 Green SM, Nakamura R, Johnson NE. Ketamine sedation for paediatric procedures: part one, a prospective series. *Ann Emerg Med* 1990;**19**:1024–32.
48 Smith JA, Santer LJ. Respiratory arrest following intramuscular ketamine injection in a 4-year old child. *Ann Emerg Med* 1993;**22**:613–5.
49 Hickey PR, Hansen DD, Cramolini GM, Vincent RN, Lang P. Pulmonary and systemic hemodynamic responses to ketamine in infants with normal and elevated pulmonary vascular resistance. *Anesthesiology* 1985;**62**:287–93.
50 Friesen RH, Henry DB. Cardiovascular changes in preterm neonates receiving isoflurane, halothane, fentanyl and ketamine. *Anesthesiology* 1986;**64**:238–42.
51 Friesen RH, Thieme RE, Honda AT, Morrison JE Jr. Changes in anterior fontanel pressure in preterm neonates receiving isoflurane, halothane, fentanyl or ketamine. *Anesth Analg* 1987;**66**:431–4.

4 Procedure related pain control

In patient care, the term "procedure" usually implies an intrusive or invasive action carried out by a clinician or nurse, with the patient awake more often than asleep, whereas an "operation" implies a surgical procedure, during which the patient is usually asleep. This chapter and the next are concerned with procedure related pain; operation induced pain is discussed in Chapter 6.

Procedures are often painful or undignified or both. They often have to be repeated, so it is important to provide optimal treatment on the first occasion, otherwise the child may come to dread future procedures; indeed, the child's fear is often the major problem to address. To control any pain caused and help the child, pharmacological and non-pharmacological methods should be used. For major procedures requiring powerful analgesia or sedation, an anaesthetist should be present as well as the paediatrician, nurse or surgeon undertaking the procedure.

We shall describe here some common problems with procedures and discuss their management.

VENOUS OR ARTERIAL CANNULATION

Venous or arterial cannulation is the most common inpatient procedure performed on children in hospital, but is mostly delegated to the least experienced doctors. This issue requires attention and debate.

Use of a topical anaesthetic (EMLA or Ametop; see page 33) is essential before elective cannulation.[1,2] The management of emergency cannulation is a major cause for concern, but alternative means of pain relief include: an ice cube inside the finger of a plastic glove (applied for 1 min); intradermal infiltration of local anaesthetic (1% buffered lignocaine) using a 29 gauge needle (as with dental procedures);[3] use of a topical refrigerant anaesthetic;[4] and Entonox oxide.[5]

To gain entry to the vein or artery in difficult cases, a Seldinger technique using a 24 gauge (blue) needle and short "neonatal" guidewire 0·012 inch in diameter (Microvena) can be used. When the fine wire is in place the site of entry can be infiltrated with local anaesthetic (1% buffered lignocaine) and the largest cannula appropriate to the size of the vein inserted over the wire.

In some children where prolonged intravenous therapy is needed, for example, meningitis in a preschool child, and there is frequent failure of peripheral venous access, a central venous line may reduce suffering (as a peripherally inserted long line or directly into the femoral or internal jugular vein).

THE FRACTIOUS CHILD

A common problem is the fractious child who is not hypoxaemic but beyond reasoning and non-pharmacological intervention. Some form of sedative may be required to enable the procedure to be carried out. If the child is already in pain and there is no vascular access, then oral or rectal codeine or morphine may be required. If the pain is severe, or the procedure is likely to cause severe pain, and there is no vascular access then subcutaneous diamorphine or intramuscular ketamine may be useful. Ketamine should only be given under the supervision of an experienced anaesthetist. If there is vascular access, intravenous morphine is appropriate. When opioid drugs or ketamine are given parenterally, professionals experienced in airway management and respiratory support must be immediately available when the drug is first given and throughout its use. Adequate respiratory and airway monitoring is essential.

If the child is not in pain but anxious, a sedative drug may be sufficient. If vascular access is available, a small dose of rapidly acting intravenous midazolam (see page 39) may be most helpful, as any adverse effects can be treated with flumazenil. Dose increments produce their effects almost immediately, so the accumulation that occurs with less rapidly acting drugs is avoided. When intravenous midazolam is given, professionals experienced in airway management and respiratory support must be immediately available at all times, and adequate respiratory and airway monitoring undertaken. If vascular access is not available then oral or rectal chloral hydrate (see page 39) can be given but its action can be slow in onset and is of long duration. Oral or intranasal midazolam may be preferable because of its more rapid and shorter duration of action.

Restlessness and agitation can be signs of hypoxaemia, and under this circumstance sedation or analgesia should not be given until the cause of hypoxaemia has been determined and treated. An anaesthetist or paediatrician experienced in advanced airway management should be present as sedation or analgesia is then administered.

RESTRAINT OF CHILDREN

When and how children should be restrained to permit essential procedures to be undertaken is a difficult subject. We do not believe that devices such as straitjackets should ever be used in these circumstances. We suggest that if restraint is required a parent should be consulted. He or she may sanction the degree of restraint required or, if they consider this inappropriate, request that the child be sedated or anaesthetised; their wishes should be respected. If an older child (say, over 8 years of age), refuses a procedure, and has been appraised of all the options, consider giving a general anaesthetic or intravenous opioid, after appropriate sedative premedication given orally, nasally or intramuscularly.

When a child too young to be reasoned with is undergoing hospital care, it is common sense to prevent him or her removing essential invasive equipment such as an arterial catheter or endotracheal tube. Straight arm splints may be useful here as well as good local fixation; however, splints should be used only when it is certain that analgesia is adequate.

NON-DRUG MEASURES

The value of non-pharmacological interventions in preparing children for invasive procedures is well established; they include play, the learning of relaxation techniques and cognitive rehearsal.

REFERENCES

1 Maunuksela EL, Korpela R. Double blind valuation of a lignocaine–prilocaine cream (EMLA) in children. *Br J Anaesth* 1986;**58**:1242–5.
2 Arts SE, Abu-Saad HH, Champion GD, *et al.* Age-related response to lidocaine–prilocaine (EMLA) emulsion and effect of music distraction on the pain of intravenous cannulation. *Pediatrics* 1994;**93**:797–801.
3 Klein EJ, Shugerman RP, Leigh-Taylor K, Schneider C, Portscheller D, Koepsell T. Buffered lidocaine: analgesia for intravenous line placement in children. *Pediatrics* 1995;**95**:709–12.
4 Abbott K, Fowler-Kerry S. The use of a topical refrigerant anesthetic to reduce injection pain in children. *J Pain Sympt Man* 1995;**10**:584–90.
5 Henderson JM, Spence DG, Komocar LM, Bonn GE, Stenstrom RJ. Administration of nitrous oxide to paediatric patients provides analgesia for venous cannulation. *Anesthesiology* 1990;**72**:269–71.

5 Procedures in the emergency department

When a child attends an accident and emergency department, the sequence of events should be triage, assessment and treatment.

TRIAGE

Pain assessment should be part of the immediate triage. Severe pain should be triaged highly, requiring at best immediate attention and at worst attention within a few minutes.

Assessment

The severity of pain can be assessed by inference, observation and use of a self report scale (see pages 11 and 96).

Treatment

Immediate treatment should comprise attention to the child's environment, supportive measures and pharmacological management of pain.

Environment

The environment should be as non-threatening and non-clinical as possible. Encourage parents to remain with their child (see page 36).

Supportive measures

The likely diagnosis, proposed treatment and priority of pain relief should be explained to child and parents. In many instances of trauma, immobilisation by splints or slings applied without moving the affected part can effect immediate physical pain relief. Any movement should be preceded by pharmacological pain relief. Parents should be encouraged to interact positively with their child by holding, stroking, touching and talking to him or her as appropriate.

Pharmacological pain control

Children in severe pain, for example, because of major trauma, femoral fracture, significant burns, displaced or comminuted fractures should receive intravenous morphine at an initial dose of 100 microgram/kg infused over 5 min (longer in infants). A further dose can be given after 5–10 min if sufficient analgesia is not achieved. The patient's pulse rate, rhythm and oxygen saturation should be monitored using pulse oximetry and electrocardiography. An anaesthetist or paediatrician experienced in advanced airway management should be immediately available if required.

There is often concern about giving morphine to a patient with major injury who may have an undetected head injury. Such a patient could lose consciousness secondary to the head injury. However, if the patient is conscious and in pain, the presence of a potential head injury is not a contraindication to giving morphine. An analgesic dose is not necessarily significantly sedative: and if the child's conscious level deteriorates, the clinician's first action should be to assess airway, breathing and circulation with cervical spine control, intervening where appropriate. In the case of concern that morphine may have caused a diminution of conscious level, intravenous naloxone (see page 27) can reverse the opioid contribution.

Femoral nerve block   In the common situation where a patient has femoral shaft fracture and a possible head injury (for example, after a road traffic accident), a femoral nerve block is usually effective. The patient is placed supine with the femur in abduction and the groin exposed. The groin is swab cleaned with antiseptic solution, and the femoral artery identified. The femoral nerve lies immediately lateral to the artery. Using a 2 ml syringe and a 25 gauge needle, infiltrate the skin just lateral to the artery with 1% lignocaine. Aspirate the syringe frequently to ensure that the needle is not in a vessel. Using a 21 gauge needle, inject bupivacaine 0·25% (maximum dose in any 6 h = 2·5 mg/kg) around the nerve, taking care not to puncture the artery or vein and using a "fanning" technique. The anaesthetised area includes the upper aspect of the thigh, the medial aspect of the leg and the periosteum of the femur. Analgesia should be achieved before the patient goes for radiography.

If the child is too distressed to proceed and sedation is unsuccessful, a general anaesthetic may be appropriate.

Fasting the patient   Fasting guidelines need to be observed before all procedures involving sedation or powerful analgesia. However, it has to be recognised that when a painful procedure has to be undertaken as an emergency these guidelines may not always be possible. Under the latter circumstances the assistance of an experienced anaesthetist will be required.

- Food/milk/formula feed: nothing for 6 h
- Breast milk: nothing for 4 h
- Clear fluids (water, dextrose, diluted clear fruit juice (no particulate matter), other soft drinks): stop for 2–3 h before sedation or general anaesthesia.

Fasting is not required when only local anaesthesia and/or Entonox are used without additional sedatives or opioids. Remember that gastric emptying may be delayed after trauma and in patients receiving opioids. If in doubt about the starvation time, give only clear fluids.

Entonox   (see page 30) can be used for emergency pain relief, but is not appropriate for continuing pain relief. It is best used as an additional analgesic for short periods of increased pain, such as during the application of slings and supports, while moving the patient or during positioning for radiography.

PROCEDURES IN THE EMERGENCY DEPARTMENT

First the clinician must decide if the planned procedure is necessary. Could the laceration be closed with glue or Steri-strips rather than stitches? Will the blood test following the venepuncture really alter the patient's management?

A child who repeatedly experiences a procedure or painful problem, for example, sickle cell episodes, will almost certainly tell you the method of pain relief he or she prefers. This does not, however, preclude improving the child's pain relief by using new techniques or drugs.

The degree and length of analgesia necessary will depend on the type of procedure. A discussion with the parents and child should include an explanation of the reason, mechanics and expected outcome of the procedure or investigation. Additionally, the child's coping mechanisms can be explored.

Some examples . . .

- A teenager presents with an airgun pellet buried in the subcutaneous tissues of the left thigh. He has attended unaccompanied.

He is listening to his favourite pop group on his personal stereo. A femoral nerve block provides complete analgesia for the procedure.

- A distressed 4-year-old requires suturing of a facial laceration. His mother says he is frightened of needles.

The child is sedated with oral midazolam (500 microgram/kg). In the treatment room his oxygen saturation is monitored. He is conscious but sleepy. While local anaesthetic (buffered 1% lignocaine at body temperature) is inserted using a 29 gauge needle, his mother shows him pictures in a pop-up book. While the sutures are placed, to discourage restlessness, she reads a favourite story. The child remains in the accident and emergency department for 2 h after the procedure, while he recovers from the sedation. He goes home with a bravery certificate.

- A 6-year-old with 15% burns on arms and chest is having a dressing changed. He has an intravenous cannula in place. He has received oral ibuprofen (4–10 mg/kg depending on his pain history).

With his mother, the boy watches a cartoon video. His mother holds, strokes, touches and talks to him throughout. Intravenous morphine (100 microgram/kg) is given just before the dressings are taken down.

In the absence of an intravenous cannula, Entonox could be used here.

6 Managing operation induced pain

There are two elements in the control of operation induced pain: preoperative and postoperative management.

PREOPERATIVE PAIN MANAGEMENT

Preoperative management comprises assessment of the child and his or her family, and establishment of a pain control plan.

Patient and family assessment

The assessment should include a history of previous painful experiences and the child's response to them. Questions to ask parents and also to discuss with an older child include:

- What sort of painful things have happened to your child in the past?
- How does your child usually react to sudden pain? Is there a different reaction to pain of a longer duration?
- Does your child tell you (or others) if he or she is in pain?
- What does your child do to get relief from pain?
- Which of these actions appear to work the best?
- Do you use pain relieving medicine at home? If so, what do you use? How do you give your child pain relieving medicine?
- Is there anything else we should know about your child and pain, or about any previous family experience of operations?

Pain control plan

The steps to consider are premedication, induction of anaesthesia and the use of analgesia during surgery.

Premedication

For premedication consider:

- EMLA or Ametop for intravenous cannula placement
- An oral sedative (such as oral midazolam 500 microgram/kg, maximum dose 15 mg)
- An oral analgesic loading dose of paracetamol (15 mg/kg) or ibuprofen (4–10 mg/kg) depending on the nature of the operation.

There is evidence that premedication with an analgesic/anti-inflammatory drug can reduce postoperative pain. Anaesthetists are increasingly using analgesics rather than sedatives for premedication and the move towards more day surgery is relevant to this issue.

- **Warning.** In the presence of upper airway obstruction that is constant (as in micrognathia) or sleep-related (as in adenotonsillar hypertrophy), sedatives (even those given orally) may produce dangerous airway obstruction. They should be omitted.

Induction of anaesthesia

Parents should be asked to stay during induction, unless their anxiety is likely to aggravate the child. The presence of a parent may also avoid the need for sedative premedication.

Analgesia

For analgesia during surgery, options include:

- Opioids or NSAIDs, which can reduce postoperative pain
- Establishing nerve or spinal cord blocks
- Wound infiltration with bupivacaine 0·25% (maximum dose 2·5 mg/kg)
- Use of local or regional anaesthesia as part of the overall strategy, unless there is a specific contraindication.

Prophylactic anti-emetics may be given at the end of the operation, when opioids are part of the pain control plan (for example, ondansetron or cyclizine; see page 27).

POSTOPERATIVE PAIN MANAGEMENT

Analgesia should be provided before postoperative pain becomes established. Use safe and effective doses of opioids, and adjunctive analgesics to gain "opioid sparing" effects. Avoid intramuscular injections.

Assess the child regularly, check the response and reassess. Children most at risk of uncontrolled pain are those with limited or absent verbal ability.

If the pain is out of proportion to the surgical trauma, consider a surgical complication and arrange reassessment of the child by surgeons. Always take a holistic approach to the child.

If the child is asleep, assume that the pain is acceptable—do not wake him or her up to make an assessment, but check regularly. If the child is awake and lying quietly, do not assume that he or she is comfortable without enquiring.

Developing a pain control plan

An individual pain control plan should be developed for each child, based on a framework that reflects the needs of both child and family.

Framework

The elements that should guide a pain control plan are:

- Willingness and ability of the child to cooperate with the pain assessment
- Existing pain relief needs, identified from the preoperative assessment
- Altered pain relief needs, as a result of admission to hospital or the disease or illness identified
- Selection of appropriate analgesic technique(s)
- Education about specific analgesic technique(s) when necessary
- Coordination of care and analgesia.

Implementing the plan

Implementing the plan of care again requires assessment, to ensure that the care delivered meets the child's and family's needs, and is a systematic approach:

- Is the analgesia effective?
- If there is a failure of analgesia:
  — is there a technical fault?
  — is a cannula misplaced?
  — is there a syringe pump malfunction?
  — are drug doses too small or too infrequent?
  — is a supplementary method or drug needed to control pain?
  — is the chosen method or drug appropriate? Should it be changed?

— has the pain outlasted its treatment? Has a local anaesthetic block worn off?

— is pain very severe and out of proportion? Is surgical re-assessment necessary?

— are non-pharmacological pain management techniques being used? Would they be valuable?

— is the reason for failed pain control a problem such as a full bladder in a child with impaired consciousness?

- If analgesia is satisfactory, are side effects present? If they are, how affected is the child by them?

Observations

The nature and frequency of observations are largely dictated by the child's condition, the overall goal of therapy and by the type of analgesic intervention used.

Evaluation

Evaluating and documenting the efficacy of the pain control plan is the final and crucial stage of the process. For children who have previously suffered uncontrolled pain, or for those with a medical or surgical condition that is likely to produce long term pain, a comprehensive evaluation may save valuable time when formulating care plans in the future, and prevent unnecessary distress to the child and family.

PARENT INFORMATION

Parents can be provided with information leaflets about their child's treatment. Examples for the parents of children who are undergoing treatment with morphine or an epidural anaesthetic are shown in Appendices E and F, courtesy of the Pain Relief Service, The Royal Hospital for Sick Children, Glasgow.

Management of postoperative nausea and vomiting[1] (PONV)

Nausea and vomiting may occur after surgery. Children at high risk of postoperative nausea and vomiting (PONV) are those:

- Undergoing otoplasty, adenotonsillectomy, strabismus repair and abdominal surgery
- With a history of PONV
- With a history of motion sickness
- Who are anxious or distressed or both
- Undergoing emergency procedures
- Who are mobilised early after their operation.

Anaesthetic techniques can be modified to reduce the incidence of PONV. For example:

- Use of newer inhalational agents such as sevoflurane
- Use of combined intraoperative analgesic techniques (for example, NSAIDs plus wound infiltration with local anaesthetics)
- Less use of opioids as premedication
- Avoidance of deep volatile anaesthesia
- Less use of prolonged fasting.

The prophylactic use, before or during surgery, of the new type 3 serotonin receptor antagonists (for example, ondansetron, 100 microgram/kg orally or intravenously to a maximum single dose of 8 mg) may also prevent or reduce PONV.

REFERENCES

1 Paxton D. Treating post operative nausea in children. *Hospital Update* 1996;**22**: 428–30.

7 Managing pain in the neonate

Most studies, some controlled, have shown that neonates, whether premature or full term, react to pain.[1,2] It is impossible to know what exactly they feel. However, a response to the insertion of needles has been demonstrated in the human fetus,[3] suggesting that this is another area for concern in terms of pain control.[4-7]

Clinical observation of neonates during "painful procedures" shows withdrawal movements, squirming, cardiovascular and respiratory changes, facial expressions, and crying, all of which suggest pain.[8] A study of neonates undergoing circumcision without analgesia or anaesthesia (the majority) suggested a subsequent long lasting reduction in pain threshold.[9] There can be no justification for not giving adequate analgesia or anaesthesia or both to neonates (or older children) undergoing this procedure.

Infants can easily be forced to endure suffering. Infants cry for many reasons, and their response to pain may not be so explicit or distressing to professionals as that expressed by an older child. Analgesia should not be withheld for fear of side effects, which the carer may be afraid of or insufficiently skilled to deal with. In these circumstances the carer should seek and be able to obtain the appropriate assistance.

Neonates are more sensitive to opioid drugs. If they need these drugs to control pain then they must be given and measures taken to deal with side effects, including assisted ventilation if required. It has to be accepted, however, that there is little known about the possible long term effects of opioids on the developing nervous system.

THE ADMINISTRATION OF ANALGESICS AND SEDATIVES TO THE NEONATE

Neonates, by virtue of their small size, inevitably require very small doses of drugs. In preparing and administering a dose or infusion, particularly of controlled drugs, it is essential that two qualified members of the nursing and/or medical staff check the prescription, dose, formulation and dilution before it is given to the patient. All parenterally given agents should be regarded as high risk since errors may produce immediate adverse or even fatal effects.

This is particularly important when, for example, morphine is being given to a neonate. The original ampoule of morphine contains at its lowest concentration 10 mg in 1 ml (that is 10,000 microgram in 1 ml). Dilution of this powerful solution can be potentially dangerous if great care is not taken. We recommend that hospital pharmacies prepare or obtain specially made up solutions of morphine for use in neonates (perhaps containing 1,000 microgram in 1 ml).

GENERAL ANAESTHESIA

Adequate general anaesthesia, additionally using opioids when needed, should usually be given for all surgical procedures on neonates. In the very preterm infant there may be an increased risk of postoperative apnoea after endotracheal general anaesthesia. The risk of this may be reduced, although not eliminated, by the use of regional anaesthesia alone.[10,11]

LOCAL ANAESTHESIA

Local anaesthetics must be used when they would be used in an older child undergoing the same procedure. However, neonates are more likely to exhibit local anaesthetic toxicity. This is because they have a lower plasma protein binding capacity for local anaesthetic drugs (as they have lower concentrations of both plasma albumin and alpha-1-acid glycoprotein) and also a lower affinity for these drugs.[12] As a result, the circulating concentrations of free drug, which cause toxicity, are higher. Reduced clearance (elimination half lives are increased two to three fold in the neonate) means the drugs can accumulate on repeated dosing or when given by infusion. In addition, the neonatal blood–brain barrier and myocardium are immature and more susceptible to local anaesthetic toxicity. Thus for lignocaine, 2·5 microgram/ml is a toxic blood level in neonates, compared to 5·0 microgram/ml in adults. Fortunately, neonates probably need smaller doses of local anaesthetics, because neonatal nerve fibres are smaller.[13]

Skin surface anaesthesia

The neonatal skin is immature and allows significant absorption of topical local anaesthetic.[14] The local anaesthetic EMLA cream does not have a product licence for use in infants. Metabolism of one of the constituents of EMLA cream, prilocaine, gives rise to oxidants to which neonates are more susceptible, because of their reduced concentration of methaemoglobin reductase. However, in one study in preterm infants EMLA reduced pain but was not shown to produce methaemoglobinaemia. This latter study did not include extremely preterm individuals who have the most immature skin and undergo the most procedures requiring surface anaesthesia.[15] EMLA is not appropriate for heel prick sampling because it induces vasoconstriction and fails to induce adequate analgesia.[16]

Topical amethocaine does not carry the risk of methaemoglobinaemia associated with prilocaine, but is not currently licensed for neonates.

Local anaesthesia by infiltration

To provide analgesia for a chest drain, for example, infiltrate 0·5% lignocaine at a maximum dose of 3 mg/kg in any 4 h period (see pages 32 and 34).

Regional anaesthesia and nerve blocks

Regional anaesthesia and nerve blocks are valuable techniques, but remember that neonates are at greater risk of toxicity from local anaesthetic drugs. For a neonate the maximum dose of bupivacaine (without adrenaline) in 6 h is 2 mg/kg. The maximum dose of lignocaine (without adrenaline) in 4 h is 3 mg/kg.

The caudal approach to the epidural space is preferable in neonates and a catheter may be advanced to the middle dermatome of the surgical wound, even when this is in the lumbar or thoracic region.[17] Spinal (subarachnoid, intrathecal) blocks can also be used but have a very short duration of action.

Systemic analgesia

Pain control with opioid drugs minimises adverse cardiovascular and metabolic responses to surgery, blunts harmful increases in pulmonary vascular resistance during tracheal suction, reduces hypoxaemia[18] and improves outcome in premature infants undergoing major operations. In the newly intubated neonate, bronchospasm and increased airway secretions in response to insertion of a plastic endotracheal airway may be dangerous and could be made worse by inadequate analgesia (D Southall, N Morton, personal observations).

However, neonates are more prone to the side effects of opioids, particularly respiratory depression, and when using these drugs, professionals experienced in airway management and respiratory support in this age group must be immediately available at all times. Adequate respiratory and airway monitoring must be undertaken.

ANALGESIA IN NEONATES RECEIVING VENTILATORY SUPPORT

When a neonate needs ventilatory support, opioids do not cause respiratory problems; indeed, they may help to prevent adverse responses to assisted ventilation.

Morphine[18-24]

Morphine has an elimination half life of 6–20 h in neonates, compared to 3–4 h in infants from 1–6 months of age. A loading dose of 100–200 microgram, as in older children, is therefore safe but may act for an unpredictably longer time. It is more likely, therefore, in the neonate, that subsequent doses will accumulate with the potential for unwanted side effects such as seizures. The loading dose should also be given more slowly: over 15–30 min. Most units maintain neonates with an intravenous infusion of 10–15 microgram/kg/h of morphine.

Morphine may delay gastric emptying and decrease intestinal motility, and may sometimes cause a significant fall in blood pressure. Blood pressure should be monitored closely when giving morphine to neonates, particularly those of extremely low birth weight.[25]

Ideally morphine should be discontinued before stopping assisted ventilation. However, in practice, particularly when long standing opioids have been needed, extubation can be concurrent with, or precede, final discontinuation of morphine.

Fentanyl

Fentanyl has a shorter duration of action than morphine and is useful during and after operations. However, it is less appropriate for general neonatal intensive care. The half life of fentanyl varies from 6–23 h in the neonate. Cardiovascular stability will usually remain with an analgesic dose of 20 microgram/kg (given over 15–30 min). Some infants may need a larger initial dose but it takes longer to eliminate than in adults. The subsequent infusion rate of fentanyl is 1–5 microgram/kg/h. Some infants develop a reduced chest wall compliance (see page 25).

58

Diamorphine

Diamorphine[26–28] is widely used in neonatal intensive care. Small but significant falls in blood pressure and heart rate may occur, but do not appear to cause clinical problems. A significant fall in respiratory rate may help synchronisation of the infant's breathing with the ventilator.

A loading dose of 50 microgram/kg is recommended, with a subsequent constant infusion at a rate of 15 microgram/kg/h.

ANALGESIA IN NEONATES NOT RECEIVING VENTILATORY SUPPORT

Morphine is a less suitable analgesic for neonates not needing assisted ventilation.

Non-opioid drugs

Codeine phosphate

Codeine phosphate 500 microgram/kg every 4 h can be given orally or rectally (2 mg and 6 mg suppositories can be halved). Codeine should not be used where there are gastrointestinal signs or symptoms, and should never be given intravenously. If more than one dose is needed, monitor respiration and oxygen saturation.

Oral paracetamol

Oral paracetamol is well absorbed from the upper small bowel within 60 min if gastric emptying is not delayed. It is available as a suspension (120 mg/5 ml); the loading dose is 10–20 mg/kg and the maintenance dose 10–15 mg/kg. The maximum daily dose is 60 mg/kg/24 h, and the dosing interval should be no less than 4 h. Do not give the maximum daily dose of paracetamol for more than 72 h.

Rectal paracetamol

Rectal paracetamol is poorly and slowly (90–120 min) absorbed from the rectum and therefore represents a slow-release form of paracetamol. Use a slightly larger loading dose and longer dosing interval than for oral paracetamol. Suppositories available contain 30 mg and 60 mg. The loading dose is 20 mg/kg and the maintenance dose 15 mg/kg. The maximum daily dose is 60 mg/kg, and the dosing intervals should be no less than 6 h. Do not give the maximum daily dose for more than 72 h.

Paracetamol doses above these levels do not give additional analgesia.

NSAIDs

NSAIDs may be more toxic in the neonatal period—hepatic, cardiac (fluid retention), renal, intestinal and platelet problems have been recorded. They are not licensed for use under 1 year of age. Careful consideration is therefore required before using them in the neonate. Ibuprofen can be used in a dose of 4 mg/kg every 6–8 h.

Morphine infusion

For a non-ventilated neonate, morphine infusion should be given only with very close monitoring in the intensive care unit.

A loading dose similar to that given to ventilated infants should be used, but perhaps given more slowly (over 30–60 min). Subsequent infusions should be given in doses that control the pain but with very close monitoring of conscious level, respiratory pattern, oxygen saturation and lung volume.

USE OF SEDATIVES IN THE NEONATE

Sedatives used in the neonate[29] include midazolam and chloral hydrate.

Midazolam

Midazolam[30] is a short-acting benzodiazepine sedative. It is not an analgesic. It should only be used in an intensive care unit with close monitoring.

In the neonate receiving analgesics (for example, a morphine infusion) midazolam may be useful in reducing the doses required and in assisting with procedures such as reintubation and the insertion of a chest drain (the latter with the addition of a local anaesthetic).

The loading dose of midazolam is 100–200 microgram/kg over 1 h. This can be followed by an intravenous infusion of 100 microgram/kg/h but this should be reduced when using morphine (60 microgram/kg/h above 33 weeks' gestation and 30 microgram/kg/h at and below 33 weeks' gestation).

When used with fentanyl, midazolam may produce hypotension.[31]

Midazolam is not recommended for long term use (more than 72 h), as increasing blood levels from poor glucuronidation may lead to dystonic posturing and an encephalopathic illness. Choreoathetosis and drowsiness have been reported 1–2 days after treatment has ended.[32]

Chloral hydrate

Chloral hydrate has been given orally in a dose of 75 mg/kg to neonates undergoing imaging.[33]

PAIN CONTROL DURING PROCEDURES

A sugar dummy, coated with 2 ml of 25–50% sucrose and given for 2 min before the procedure, can be helpful.[34-38] Breast feeding during procedures may be equally as valuable.[39] However, in babies who are poor feeders, care must be taken not to associate feeding activities with pain. If recurrent invasive procedures are needed, the use of a distraction strategy relating to feeding may be detrimental.

When a procedure is undertaken the physical movements of the baby may get out of control. In all cases comfort and containment (swaddling) should be provided by a parent or a nurse.[40,41]

For heel pricks the Autolet, Glucolet or Tenderfoot devices are less painful than manual skin puncture.[42,43] The Tenderfoot is said to produce a better blood yield.[44] EMLA should not be used because it produces vasoconstriction and the heel does not bleed well.[16] Oral sucrose can also help.[45]

Circumcision without general anaesthesia is not recommended, but if so performed should be carried out with regional local anaesthetic. A penile nerve block using lignocaine (which must not include a vasoconstrictor) can be a good way of providing this.[46]

For arterial or venous puncture or insertion of arterial or venous catheters

Apply EMLA cream 30–60 min before the procedure, using only a pea sized quantity of gel. The skin surface barrier is less established in the neonate than in the older infant or child, so there is a risk of greater absorption of the local anaesthetic.

The non-vasoconstricting local anaesthetic cream Ametop may be useful, but, like EMLA, is not yet licensed for neonates.

For suprapubic aspiration or lumbar puncture

Use EMLA cream[47,48] or a local infiltration with 0·5–1·0% lignocaine[49,50] (maximum dose = 3 mg/kg). Local infiltration does not make lumbar punctures more difficult to perform.[49]

GENERAL MEASURES TO IMPROVE HOSPITAL CARE FOR INFANTS

Attempts should be made to provide a baby friendly environment[51] and the infant should be kept warm and the nappy area clean and dry.

Contact with parents, such as cuddles, singing, feeding (especially breast feeding) and "kangaroo care"[52] should be encouraged.

Gentle massage by relatives, nurses or doctors may be soothing for the baby, and there should be minimal noise, particularly from monitors. Intense lighting should also be avoided. Do not disrupt sleep unless it is essential. Infants should sleep on a comfortable surface, such as a sheepskin.

When frequent blood sampling is required, central venous and arterial lines should be used to avoid needling of the skin. If an operation is performed, such lines should be inserted prophylactically under the general anaesthesia and then securely fixed to avoid postoperative displacement. Repeated and unnecessary examinations should be avoided.

ASSESSMENT OF NEONATAL PAIN

Assessment of pain may be very difficult in the very preterm infant.[53-55] It is less easy for very immature infants to demonstrate responses such as crying, facial grimacing or withdrawal movements. This is not because they do not suffer the effects of pain. Moreover, physiological changes, such as an increased heart rate, increased blood pressure and decreased oxygen saturation, are not specific for pain.

If in doubt about the presence of pain, for example, in necrotising enterocolitis, which may come on gradually and would be expected from the pathophysiology to produce severe pain, give an analgesic such as codeine or morphine.

It is important to assess the effect of an intervention on the pattern of behavioural and physiological changes. If they do not improve, then the intervention may have been inadequate or the original observations may not have been the result of pain.

Neonatal pain assessment scores

The following basic observations provide indicators of pain that can be scored and charted.

- Alertness: *asleep/awake*

If asleep, stop assessment. If awake, proceed.

- Crying: *not crying versus crying*
- Posture: *relaxed versus moving, especially limb flexion*
- Facial expression: *neutral versus distressed (brow bulging*, eyes closed)*

* Brow bulging during sleep may also indicate pain.

Table 7.1   *CRIES:*[56] *a score for the measurement of postoperative pain in neonates who are not intubated or paralysed. HR, heart rate, BP, blood pressure*

Parameter	Score*		
	0	1	2
Crying	None	High pitched	Inconsolable
Requires O_2 to keep oxygen saturation $\geqslant 95\%$	No	< 30%	> 30%
Increased vital signs	HR and BP equal to or below preoperative values	HR and BP increased <20% over preoperative values	HR and BP increased >20% over preoperative values
Expression	None	Grimace	Grimace/grunt
Sleepless	No	Wakes at frequent intervals	Constantly awake

* For more details on coding see original reference.[56]

- Physical changes: *constant heart rate, normal breathing pattern and oxygen saturation versus increased heart rate, irregular breathing, oxygen saturation reduced, increased blood pressure, pallor*

More useful is a dynamic assessment, where improvement in behavioural and physiological changes is sought in response to comforting, analgesia or sedation. Table 7·1 shows a scoring system that works well in all but the very preterm or sedated/paralysed infants. The higher the score the greater the pain. Disadvantages of such a system are that oxygenation is affected by many other factors, and the taking of blood pressure measurements may upset the baby.

Liverpool infant distress score (LIDS)[57]

The behaviour of neonates has been analysed using video recordings to produce an objective scoring system indicative of pain-suffering.

REFERENCES

1 Anand KJS Hickey PR. Pain and its effects in the human neonate and fetus. *N Engl J Med* 1987;**317**:1321–9.
2 Fitzgerald M, Millard C, McIntosh N. Cutaneous hypersensitivity following peripheral tissue damage in newborn infants and its reversal with topical anaesthesia. *Pain* 1989;**39**:31–6.
3 Giannakoulopoulos X, Sepulveda W, Kourtis P, *et al.* Fetal plasma cortisol and β-endorphin response to intrauterine needling. *Lancet* 1994;**344**:77–81.
4 Derbyshire SWG, Furedi A. Do fetuses feel pain? *BMJ* 1996;**313**:795.
5 Glover V, Fisk N. We don't know; better to err on the safe side from mid-gestation. *BMJ* 1996;**313**:796.

6 Szawarski Z. Probably no pain in the absence of "self". *BMJ* 1996;**313**:796–7.
7 Glover V, Giannakoulopoulos X. Stress and pain in the fetus. *Baillière's Clin Paediatr* 1995;**3**:495–510.
8 Craig KD, Whitfield MF, Grunau RVE, *et al.* Pain in the preterm neonate: behavioural and physiological indices. *Pain* 1993;**52**:287–99.
9 Taddio A, Goldbach M, Ipp M, *et al.* Effect of neonatal circumcision on pain responses during vaccination in boys. *Lancet* 1995;**345**:291–2.
10 Sartorelli KH, Abajian JC, Kreutz JM, Vane DW. Improved outcome utilizing spinal anesthesia in high risk neonates. *J Pediatr Surg* 1992;**27**:1022–5.
11 Krane EJ, Haberkern CM, Jacobson LE. Postoperative apnea, bradycardia and oxygen desaturation in formerly premature infants: prospective comparison of spinal and general anesthesia. *Anesth Analg* 1995;**80**:7–13.
12 Eyres RL. Local anaesthetic agents in infancy. *Pediatr Anaesth* 1995;**5**:213–8.
13 Duron B, Khater-Boidin J. Electrophysiological aspects of peripheral nervous system development. *Neurophysiologie Clinique* 1992;**22**:225–47.
14 Barrett DA, Rutter N. Percutaneous lignocaine absorption in newborn infants. *Arch Dis Child* 1994;**71**:F122–4.
15 Taddio A, Shennan AT, Stevens B, *et al.* Safety of lidocaine-prilocaine cream in the treatment of preterm neonates. *J Paediatr* 1995;**127**:1002–5.
16 McIntosh N, van Veen L, Bramayer H. Alleviation of the pain of heel prick in preterm infants. *Arch Dis Child* 1994;**70**:F177–81.
17 Goldman LJ. Complications in regional anaesthesia. *Pediatr Anaesth* 1995;**5**: 3–9.
18 Pokela ML. Pain relief can reduce hypoxemia in distressed neonates during routine treatment procedures. *Pediatrics* 1994;**93**:379–83.
19 Quinn MW, Wild J, Dean HG, *et al.* Randomised double-blind controlled trial of effect of morphine on catecholamine concentrations in ventilated pre-term babies. *Lancet* 1993;**342**:324–7.
20 Bhat R, Chari G, Gulati A, *et al.* Pharmacokinetics of a single dose of morphine in preterm infants during the first week of life. *J Paediatr* 1990; **117**:477–81.
21 Lynn AM, Slattery JT. Morphine pharmacokinetics in early infancy. *Anesthesiology* 1987;**66**:136–9.
22 Hartley R, Levene MI. Opioid pharmacology in the newborn. *Clin Paediatr* 1991;**3**:467–94.
23 Koren G, Butt W, Chinyanga H, *et al.* Postoperative morphine infusion in newborn infants: assessment of disposition characteristics and safety. *J Pediatr* 1985;**107**:963–7.
24 Chay PC, Duffy BJ, Walker JS. Pharmacokinetic-pharmacodynamic relationships of morphine in neonates. *Clin Pharm Thera* 1992;**51**:334–42.
25 Setzer N. Anesthesia, premature infants and hypotension. *Pediatrics* 1993;**93**: 870.
26 Elias-Jones AC, Barrett DA, Rutter N, *et al.* Diamorphine infusion in the preterm neonate. *Arch Dis Child* 1991;**66**:F1155–7.
27 Rutter, Richardson. A survey of the use of analgesia in newborn intensive care. *Int J Pharm Prac* 1992;**1**:220–2.
28 Barker DP, Simpson J, Pawula M, *et al.* Randomised, double blind trial of two loading dose regimens of diamorphine in ventilated newborn infants. *Arch Dis Child* 1995;**73**:F22–6.
29 Levene MI, Quinn MW. Use of sedatives and muscle relaxants in newborn babies receiving mechanical ventilation. *Arch Dis Child* 1992;**67**:870–3.
30 Jacqz-Aigrain E, Daoud P, Burtin P, *et al.* Placebo-controlled trial of midazolam sedation in mechanically ventilated newborn babies. *Lancet* 1994;**344**:646–50.
31 Burtin P, Daoud P, Jacqz-Aigrain E, *et al.* Hypotension with midazolam and fentanyl in the newborn. *Lancet* 1991;**337**:1545–6.
32 Bergman I, Sreeves M, Buckart G, Thompson A. Reversible neurological abnormalities associated with prolonged intravenous midazolam and fentanyl administration. *J Pediatr* 1991;**119**:644–9.
33 McCarver-May DG, Kang J, Aouthmany M, *et al.* Comparison of chloral hydrate and midazolam for sedation of neonates for neuroimaging studies. *J Pediatr* 1996; **128**;4:573–6.

34 Haouari N, Wood C, Griffiths G, Levene M. The analgesic effect of sucrose in full term infants: a randomised controlled trial. *BMJ* 1995;**310**:1498–500.

35 Blass EM, Hoffmeyer LB. Sucrose as an analgesic for newborn infants. *Paediatrics* 1991;**87**:215–8.

36 Bucher HU, Moser T, Von Siebenthal K, *et al*. Sucrose reduces pain reaction to heel lancing in preterm infants: a placebo controlled randomised and masked study. *Pediatr Res* 1995;**38**:332–5.

37 Ramenghi LA, Griffith GC, Wood CM, Levene MI. Effect of non-sucrose sweet tasting solution on neonatal heel prick responses. *Arch Dis Child* 1996;**74**: F129–31.

38 Ramenghi LA, Wood CM, Griffith GC, Levene MI. Reduction of pain response in premature infants using intraoral sucrose. *Arch Dis Child* (Fetal and Neonatal Edition) 1996;**74**:F126–8.

39 Jepson C. Cuddle deprivation may have confounded experiment. *BMJ* 1995; **311**:747–8.

40 McIntosh N, van Veen L, Brameyer H. Alleviation of the pain of heel prick in preterm infants. *Arch Dis Child* 1994;**70**:F177–81.

41 Campos RG. Soothing pain-elicited distress in infants with swaddling and pacifiers. *Child Devel* 1989;**60**:781–92.

42 Harpin VA, Rutter N. Making heel pricks less painful. *Arch Dis Child* 1983;**58**: 226–8.

43 McIntosh N, van Veen L, Brameyer H. The pain of heel prick and its measurement in infants. *Pain* 1993;**52**:71–4.

44 Barker DP, Latty BW, Rutter N. Heel blood sampling in preterm infants: which technique? *Arch Dis Child* 1994;**71**:F206–8.

45 Rushforth JA, Levene MI. Effect of sucrose on crying in response to heel stab. *Arch Dis Child* 1993;**69**:388–9.

46 Maxwell LG, Yaster M, Wetzel RC, Niebyl JR. Penile nerve block for newborn circumcision. *Obstet Gynecol* 1987;**70**:415–9.

47 Kapelushnik J, Koren G, Solh H, *et al*. Evaluating the efficacy of EMLA in alleviating pain associated with lumbar puncture: comparison of open and double-blinded protocols in children. *Pain* 1990;**42**:31–4.

48 Young AC, *et al*. Lignocaine–prilocaine cream for lumbar puncture. *Lancet* 1987;**2**:1533.

49 Pinheiro JMB, Furdon S, Ochoa LF. Role of local anesthesia during lumbar puncture in neonates. *Pediatrics* 1993;**91**:379–82.

50 Porter FL, Miller JP, Cole FS, Marshall RE. A controlled clinical trial of local anesthesia for lumbar punctures in newborns. *Pediatrics* 1991;**88**:663–9.

51 Als H, Lawhon G, Brown E, *et al*. Individualized behavioural and environmental care for the very low birth weight preterm infant at high risk for bronchopulmonary dysplasia: neonatal intensive care unit and developmental outcome. *Pediatrics* 1986;**78**:1123–32.

52 Anderson GC. Current knowledge about skin-to-skin (kangaroo) care for preterm infants. *J Perinat* 1991;**11**:216–26.

53 Moorse CA, McIntosh N. Assessing analgesia of morphine and hyperalgesia of withdrawal in neonates using the flexor withdrawal reflex. Submitted for publication.

54 Grunau RVE, Craig KD. Pain expression in neonates: facial action and cry. *Pain* 1987;**28**:395–410.

55 Rushforth JA, Levene M. Behavioural response to pain in healthy neonates. *Arch Dis Child* 1994;**70**:F174–6.

56 Krechel SW, Bildner J. Cries: a new neonatal post operative pain measurement score. Initial testing of validity and reliability. *Paediatr Anaesth* 1995;**5**:53–61.

57 Horgan M, Choonara I, *et al*. Measuring pain in neonates: An objective score. *Paediatric Nursing* 1996;**8**:24–7.

8 Pain management during intensive care

When a child requires intensive care, every effort should be made to avoid the need for emergency procedures, such as intubation, by adequate monitoring and provision of airway and blood oxygenation, maintenance of lung volume and airway care. Emergency procedures are often extremely painful, dangerous to the child and represent a failure of intensive care. They should be audited. Where possible all invasive procedures should be elective.

Muscle relaxants should never be used unless the child is free of pain and sedated; avoid partial paralysis.

Intensive care staff should aim to provide an environment that is friendly to children and their families. Ideally all children should be cared for in a paediatric intensive care unit rather than in an adult unit—this is particularly important in the conscious child.

Helpful measures are as follows:

- Provide a day/night cycle (uninterrupted natural sleep can lessen the need for analgesia or sedation) and ensure minimal noise and low lighting between 8 pm and 8 am.
- Deal with emergency admissions at night away from sleeping patients.
- Set monitors to alarm audibly only when essential.
- Consider ear plugs for the child, especially when he or she is paralysed.
- Ensure frequent human input through voice, touch, music, cuddling, rocking, holding and pacifying.
- Consider distraction, play therapy, relaxation, behavioural techniques, hypnosis and aromatherapy. Such measures are particularly valuable in patients undergoing long term intensive or high dependency care.
- Provide privacy when possible.
- Watch for depression after prolonged intensive care.[1,2] Consider seeking help from a child psychiatrist, child psychologist or child psychiatric nurse.

PROLONGED INTENSIVE CARE

Difficulties arise in practice when a child's illness results in prolonged intensive care, perhaps for more than 4–6 weeks. The number of procedures endured during this time[3] and the declining effectiveness of analgesics and sedatives can result in suffering that is difficult or impossible to control. This raises moral and ethical issues that are not easy to deal with. We offer here some suggestions and comments.

The whole team of professionals involved in caring for the child—doctors, nurses, social workers, psychologists, physiotherapists—and the parents should discuss the problem, and look at all the child's needs. If the child is old enough to be involved, his or her opinion is of major importance. Often, however, the child is too young or too ill to contribute. A key point to consider when deciding to continue is that every effort must be made to ensure that all future procedures are undertaken without causing suffering. This may entail giving doses of drugs or medications that themselves have an increased risk. As the child is usually unable to consent or refuse to continue intensive care, such decisions have to be made with great care, with the wellbeing of the child as the most important factor. The feelings of parents and staff must always be secondary to this right of the child. Sometimes the advice of a specialist from another centre may assist in decision making. Rarely the hospital ethics review board or even a court may need to be approached.

INVASIVE PROCEDURES IN INTENSIVE CARE

Invasive procedures in intensive care, as in any other situation, must be preceded by an explanation and preparation of the child. Explanation, with bedside comforting measures, can reduce anxiety, as can appropriate drug therapy. For children mature enough and awake enough, explanations should include an outline of why the procedure is necessary. Children should receive appropriate personal support during the procedure from a parent, nurse, doctor or other care-giver, even if they are receiving background analgesia and sedation and particularly if they are paralysed.

Before performing an invasive procedure, always consider:

- Is the procedure essential at this time?
- Could I avoid this procedure by sampling from an indwelling arterial or central venous line?
- Would the use of non-invasive monitoring of, for example, carbon dioxide, reduce the number of procedures?

Table 8.1 *Single intravenous doses of analgesic and sedative drugs, given to cover invasive procedures or as a prelude to establishing effective infusions*

Drug	Single dose	Side effects and contraindications
Must be given only when an anaesthetist or intensivist is immediately available		
Morphine*	50–200 microgram/kg	Respiratory depression/loss of airway protective reflexes. Nausea, vomiting and possible aspiration. Hypotension
Fentanyl*	1–20 microgram/kg	As morphine. Chest wall rigidity may occur with rapid infusion therefore give over 15 min
Ketamine	1–4 mg/kg	Muscle tone maintained. Blood pressure may rise
	For 5–10 min of surgical anaesthesia give over a minimum of 60 s. For longer maintenance, give 10–45 microgram/kg/min according to response	Hallucinations and other psychotic manifestations may occur. Increased salivation and airway irritability/secretions (including laryngospasm) may occur—particularly in infants Contraindicated in hypertension and intracranial problems.
Midazolam	100–200 microgram/kg	Respiratory depression. May potentiate respiratory and cardiovascular depression of opioids. Variable duration of action in liver failure. Injection may be painful if given into peripheral vein—can cause thrombophlebitis
Propofol	2 mg/kg to 2·5 mg/kg	10% lipid emulsion preparation. Not licensed for use under 3 years of age.

* Combinations of a systemic opioid with an intravenous anti-emetic may avoid vomiting in susceptible children (see pages 27–8). Entonox may also be useful (page 30).

All invasive procedures must be preceded by adequate local and, when necessary, systemic analgesia (see Table 8.1). Specific measures are required to prevent acute rises in intracranial pressure in selected ventilated patients, for example, by a short-acting intravenous bolus of opioid.

For procedures that jeopardise airway or respiratory function such as intubation, a skilled professional able to deal with all unforeseen eventualities should be present. Usually this will be a paediatrician skilled in neonatal or paediatric intensive care or a paediatric anaesthetist. Respiratory and airway monitoring must be adequate. Every effort should be made to undertake these procedures electively, but emergencies will occur. Specialist training courses in paediatric life support techniques are invaluable for all doctors and nurses caring for children in intensive care (see Resources, page 93).

COMMON PROCEDURES

Some examples of invasive procedures and possible pain control measures are given below.

Venous or arterial cannulation
This is discussed on pages 43–44.

Insertion of a urinary catheter
Lignocaine gel 2% into the urethra should be given at least 10 min before the procedure (see page 33).

Insertion of a pleural drain
This requires infiltration of lignocaine 1% to skin and tissue, as deep as the parietal pleura. The maximum dose in any 4 h is 4 mg/kg (3 mg/kg in neonates) and the maximum single total dose 200 mg.

Allow 10 min for the full local anaesthetic effect to develop. If urgent placement is needed, as in relieving tension pneumothorax, consider needle decompression (thoracocentesis) as a life-saving measure while waiting for the local anaesthetic to act.

Suture, drain, or cannula removal
Give opioid analgesia ± midazolam as an intravenous bolus.

Airway procedures
Intubation in the neonate, infant or child whose level of consciousness is receptive to pain must be accompanied by analgesia as well as muscle relaxation. Intubation therefore requires considerable experience with drug administration as well as with the procedure itself. A skilled professional, able to deal with all unforeseen eventualities, should be present. Usually this will be a paediatrician skilled in neonatal or paediatric intensive care or a paediatric anaesthetist. Adequate respiratory and airway monitoring must be undertaken during the procedure.

Intubation may be required in four settings: rapid sequence induction, a difficult or obstructed airway, elective intubation, and replacement of an existing endotracheal tube. If only an inexperienced operator is available, then basic respiratory support involving airway opening and bag and mask ventilation should be continued until either an experienced operator is present or effective ventilation cannot be sustained without intubation.

Rapid sequence induction
When intubation is carried out as part of a rapid sequence induction, there is a risk of regurgitation and aspiration of gastric contents.

There is usually no time for premedication. The patient is pre-oxygenated, sedation/analgesia is usually given in the form of thiopentone, ketamine or propofol, paralysis is given as suxamethonium and cricoid pressure is used.

Difficult or obstructed airway

When a difficult or obstructed airway is present in a patient requiring intubation, an anaesthetist experienced in airway management in children and an ENT surgeon able, if necessary, to undertake a rigid bronchoscopy or tracheostomy must be urgently summoned. (In a specialist paediatric intensive care unit, the intensivists are often sufficiently experienced not to need a surgeon's help.) Facilities for cricothyroidotomy should also be immediately available.

The first procedure in this situation would usually be to secure the airway. Increased inspired oxygen can be provided by elephant tubing or by a face mask held close to the child, without upsetting him or her if possible. Anaesthesia can then be induced, using halothane and oxygen through the same route. Continuous positive airways pressure should be applied up to 20 cm H_2O, to maintain the airway as the child becomes unconscious; the apparatus used should be a mask and a paediatric T-piece circuit connected via an anaesthetic (Boyle's) machine, which also allows the delivery of nearly 100% oxygen via the mask.

In the child with airway obstruction or a difficult airway even mild sedatives are contraindicated. Muscle relaxants are absolutely forbidden because ventilation by bag and mask may become impossible once the relaxant takes effect. Anticipate upper airway obstruction as a possible problem in children with large heads, small lower jaws and protruding tongues, for example those with Down's syndrome.

Elective intubation

Elective intubation, where the airway is not difficult or obstructed, requires the presence of an experienced operator but not the presence of an ENT surgeon. In a child who is fractious and beyond reasoning in whom hypoxaemia is not the cause, a premedication with oral midazolam or intramuscular ketamine may be helpful (see page 39–40).

Changing an endotracheal tube

When there is an established endotracheal airway, the tube may need changing electively (for example, from an oral to a nasal tube) or as an emergency if the existing tube becomes blocked.

Elective tube change Ensure the child is receiving adequate analgesia and sedation and that an adequate dose of muscle relaxant has been given to obtain the best possible conditions for intubation. Use full cardiorespiratory monitoring throughout, and give 2–3 min ventilation with 100% oxygen before the tube change (preoxygenation). Check the size and length of the tube in place and have ready a similar tube and two others of smaller diameter (internal diameter smaller by 0·5 and 1·0 mm). Also have ready several different laryngoscopes, an intubation stylet, a flexible plastic bougie and Magill forceps, as well as working suction apparatus. Perform a laryngoscopy to ensure the anatomy of the larynx is normal and the vocal cords easily visualised. Under direct vision pass the new tube anterior to the existing tube and have an assistant remove the existing tube. Advance the new tube into the trachea, assisting its progress by rotation through 180 degrees or by using the Magill forceps. This technique is appropriate for nasal and oral intubation, and uses the existing tube and a good view of the vocal cords as landmarks for the new tube.

Where the anatomy is distorted or abnormal, changing tubes requires extreme care. A silastic or plastic bougie, suction catheter or guidewire can be passed via the existing tube and a new tube advanced over this guide using a railroading technique. This is a method for experts only and is fraught with technical hazards. Fibreoptic guided intubation techniques may be useful in specific cases, but should be undertaken only by those appropriately trained in this method.

Management of analgesia/sedation in the intubated child

Intubation usually requires background analgesia and sedation for at least 3 days. Use the minimum doses of analgesia to ensure comfort and security of the airway. Inadequate pain control in intubated patients may lead to airway injury from crying and squirming movements. (The possible relationship between pain control and airway injury needs to be investigated.)[8]

In newly intubated patients—particularly infants with peripheral lung disorders such as bronchiolitis—bronchospasm and increased airway secretions in response to the presence of a plastic endotracheal airway and endotracheal suction[4-7] can be dangerous or life threatening. These problems are made worse or even generated by inadequate analgesia, which is common in these situations because of fears of being unable to continue to ventilate the child.

Endotracheal suction

Endotracheal suction is potentially painful in the first 3 days after intubation,[9] particularly in children with tracheitis. Intubation therefore requires background analgesia and sedation for at least

Table 8.2 *Drug infusions for background analgesia and sedation*

Drug	Doses	Preparation of infusion
Morphine†	10–100 microgram/kg/h (usual upper limit = 50 microgram/kg/h) (10–20 microgram/kg/h is usually sufficient in neonates) Care in renal failure as metabolite accumulates	Use preservative free solution. 2 mg/kg made up to 50 ml in 5 or 10% glucose or 0·9% saline. Then infusion of 1 ml/h of this concentration = 40 microgram/kg/h.
Midazolam	25–250 microgram/kg/h Variable duration of action in liver failure	5 mg/kg made up to 50 ml in 5 or 10% glucose or 0·9% saline. Then infusion of 1 ml/h of this concentration = 100 microgram/kg/h.
Fentanyl	1–8 microgram/kg/h (1–4 microgram/kg/h in neonates)	Undiluted solution = 50 microgram/ml. Wt in kg × 0.08 = ml/h of undiluted solution to give 4 microgram/kg/h
Propofol*	1–4 mg/kg/h	Undiluted solution = 10 mg/ml. Wt in kg × 0.2 = ml/h of neat solution to give 2 mg/kg/h. Administer in PVC giving sets

* Not for use in those under 3 years of age or for more than 24 h. Ideally use with opioid infusion to reduce dose needed. Consider monitoring blood lipid levels.
† For example, if body wt is 5 kg, then add 2 × 5 = 10 mg of morphine to 50 ml of 5% glucose and then 1 ml/h of this solution gives the patient 40 microgram/kg/h.

3 days. If the child reacts adversely to suction, and other parameters suggest that he or she is suffering pain, then the background systemic analgesia/sedation may be inadequate (Table 8.2). Under these circumstances consider giving a short-acting bolus of an opioid (such as fentanyl) before undertaking airway toilet.

BACKGROUND ANALGESIA AND SEDATION FOR INTENSIVE CARE

Table 8·2 lists regimens for providing systemic analgesics and sedatives to children in intensive care.

All systemic analgesics and sedatives have unwanted side effects. The goal should be to use the minimum dose that leaves the child comfortable. Infusion rates should therefore be constantly adjusted to satisfy the needs of the child.

Avoid intramuscular injections by giving sedatives and analgesics intravenously or enterally.

Weaning from background infusions

Stopping background opioid or midazolam infusion can be difficult, and there is little research to guide us. Analgesia and sedation or both have to be withdrawn slowly after prolonged use.[10] Problems arise when long term infusions have resulted in physical dependency.

Signs of opioid withdrawal include agitation, abdominal pain, dysaesthesia and muscle cramps. These need to be distinguished from the pain and discomfort of the underlying problem for which long term opioids have been given.

In general, a maximum reduction in daily dosage of 10–20% per day is a practical guide for those who have received long term infusions of opioids or midazolam. Withdrawal should be guided by clinical assessment and may need to be undertaken more slowly.

Suggested approaches to weaning from a continuous infusion of opioids[11,12]

In general, patients who have been treated with low to moderate doses of opioids for <5 days can be weaned within 3–4 days. If high dose opioids have been given for >5 days, proportionally longer will be required to wean them—possibly up to 2 or 3 weeks.

During weaning close and regular clinical assessment is essential. The original drug may be used for weaning, although methadone with its longer duration of action may be preferable.

The following strategy has been suggested by Anand.[12]

1. Gradually decrease the intravenous infusion rate, initially by 20–40% and later by 10–20% of the original dose every 12–24 h.
2. Convert from intermittent doses of morphine given every 2–4 h, then to methadone given every 6 h. For methadone, an equipotent 24 h dose can be given in divided 6 hourly doses or at an initial dose of 200 microgram/kg orally or 100 microgram/kg intravenously every 6 h with progressive increases of 50 microgram/kg until signs or symptoms have resolved. It has to be recognised that significant under- or overdose is possible when changing from one opioid to another. Close observation is essential.

   It should be noted that since intravenous methadone has a slower onset of action (2 h) than other opioids the existing opioid infusion of morphine, diamorphine or fentanyl should not be stopped until at least 2 h after the first converting dose of methadone has been started intravenously.
3. After the first 24–48 h of weaning, the interval between doses of morphine or methadone can be progressively increased (to 8, then 12 then 24 hourly).
4. Methadone has, usefully, a prolonged half life and it can be discontinued after the patient is down to doses of

50–100 microgram/kg/24 h in neonates and children <4 years and to doses of 10–20 microgram/kg/24 h in older children and adolescents.
5. Morphine or methadone can be given orally or via the nasogastric tube when dose intervals have decreased to every 12 to 24 h.
6. At all stages the aim should be to keep the patient free of agitation and distress, but able to sleep and not to be excessively sedated.
7. Adjunctive drugs do not have a well defined role in weaning patients from opioids. Carefully reducing doses of opioids represents the best way of managing opioid withdrawal. Nevertheless, small doses of benzodiazepines in addition to opioids, may be useful in controlling irritability, anxiety or seizures associated with opioid withdrawal. For example, diazepam 100–300 microgram/kg every 6 h intravenously or orally, depending on the severity of the withdrawal. Patients should be closely monitored for respiratory depression and hypotension.

Midazolam is not recommended because of its short duration of action.

Clonidine orally in doses of 3–4 microgram/kg has been shown to be helpful in neonates[13] with weaning over 1–2 weeks.

Alternative approaches include short periods (less than 24 h) using propofol or ketamine infusions which can provide a break from morphine, thereby reducing dependence while maintaining adequate analgesia.

Suggested approaches to weaning from a continuous benzodiazepine infusion

This involves the use of a long-acting benzodiazepine—such as diazepam—together with other sedatives such as phenobarbitone or chloral hydrate as required. Diazepam has approximately dose for dose half of the sedative potency of midazolam. Starting doses of diazepam of 200–300 microgram/kg every 4 to 6 h (intravenously or orally) are usually sufficient unless very high doses over long time periods have been used. Careful clinical assessment and reassessments are required.

Patients given low doses can generally be weaned within 3–4 days, but those on continuous high dose infusions may require several weeks.

USE OF MUSCLE RELAXANTS IN INTENSIVE CARE

Muscle relaxants are invaluable and widely used in the treatment of critically ill children. However, they should never be used without ensuring that the patient is both pain free and sedated. Partial paralysis should be avoided.

Table 8.3 *Analgesics and sedatives given by the oral or nasogastric route (see pages 16–24)*

Drug	Doses	Side effects/ contraindications
Chloral hydrate	25–100 mg/kg Every 4–8 h as required Maximum single dose = 1 g Maximum dose in 24 h = 3 g	Contraindicated in upper airway obstruction, gastric irritation. Hypotension when given with frusemide
Codeine phosphate	0·5–1 mg/kg every 4–6 h	Do not use in renal impairment. Never give intravenously. Watch for respiratory depression, especially in neonates
Diazepam	Age 4 weeks to 1 year: 50 microgram/kg/12 h Age 1–4 years: 500 microgram/12 h Age 5–12 years: 1·0 to 1·5 mg/12 h Age 13–18 years: 2 mg/12 h	Beware respiratory depression
Diclofenac	0·5–1·5 mg/kg/12 h or up to 1 mg/kg every 8 h	Do not use if predisposition to gastric bleeding in thrombocytopenia or other coagulation abnormalities or in renal impairment. Caution in asthma.
Ibuprofen	4–10 mg/kg every 6–8 h *or* Age 1–2 years: 50 mg 3–4 times a day Age 3–7 years: 100 mg 3–4 times a day Age 8–12 years: 200 mg 3–4 times a day	Not licensed for use under 1 year of age
Morphine	200–400 microgram/kg Over 12 years 10–15 mg Every 4 h for short acting preparation	Ceiling dose depends on history of use. Respiratory depression, nausea/vomiting, pruritus, constipation, urinary retention
Paracetamol	Suspension: 120 mg/5 ml or 250 mg/5 ml (sugar free forms preferred; colorant free forms may be indicated for specific children; strawberry or banana flavours available) Tablets: 500 mg Soluble: 500 mg Loading dose: 20 mg/kg Maintenance dose: 15 mg/kg Maximum daily dose: 90 mg/kg/24 h (60 mg/kg/24 h in neonates) Dosing no more frequent than every 4 h. Do not give maximum daily dose for more than 72 h	Not in children with liver disease

(continued)

Table 8.3 *(continued)—Analgesics and sedatives given by the oral or nasogastric route*

Drug	Doses	Side effects/ contraindications
Promethazine	Age 4 weeks to 1 year: 5 mg every 12 h Age 1–5 years: 10 mg every 12 h Age 6–10 years: 20 mg every 12 h	May cause hyperexcitability
Trimeprazine	300 microgram/kg every 8 h or 250 microgram/kg every 6 h	May cause hyperexcitability

Table 8.4 *Analgesics and sedatives given rectally*

Drug	Doses	Side effects/ contraindications
Chloral hydrate	Give as enema in olive oil by syringe (100 mg/ml or 500 mg/ml) 25–100 mg/kg, every 4–8 h	Maximum safe dose in 24 h = 3 g As with oral
Paracetamol	Suppositories: 60 mg, 125 mg, 250 mg, 500 mg, 1 g Loading dose: 30 mg/kg, (20 mg/kg in neonates) Maintenance dose: 20 mg/kg (15 mg/kg in neonates) Maximum daily dose: 90 mg/kg/24 h (60 mg/kg/24 h in neonates). Dosing should be no more frequent than every 6 h. Do not give maximum daily dose for more than 72 h. Doses above these levels do not give additional analgesia.	Poorly and slowly (90–120 min) absorbed from the rectum; acts like a slow-release form of paracetamol. Need a larger loading dose and longer dosing interval than when the drug is given orally. Paracetamol is contraindicated in children with liver disease
Diclofenac	Suppositories: 12·5 mg, 25 mg, 50 mg, 100 mg, 0·5–1·0 mg/kg two or three times daily Maximum daily dose: 3 mg/kg/24 h	Not for use with gastric bleeding Cautions as for oral preparation

USE OF ENTERALLY GIVEN DRUGS

When appropriate, parenteral analgesics and sedatives should be superceded by drugs given orally or via a nasogastric tube (Table 8.3). If bowel sounds are not present then further reductions in intravenous analgesics such as opioids or discontinuation of muscle relaxants may be required before oral or nasogastric preparations can be given. However, in the meantime, drugs may be given rectally (Table 8.4). Enterally given analgesics and sedatives need to be started before systemic agents are discontinued and initially prescribed at regular intervals (every 4–6 h), and not on an "as required" basis.

REFERENCES

1 Jones C, Griffiths RD, MacMillan R, Palmer TEA. Psychological problems occurring after intensive care. *Br J Int Care* 1994;**4**:46–53.

2 Ambuel B, Hamlett KW, Marx CM, Blumer JL. Assessing distress in pediatric intensive care environments: the COMFORT scale. *J Pediatr Psychol* 1992;**17**: 95–109.

3 Southall DP, Cronin BC, Hartmann H, *et al*. Invasive procedures in children receiving intensive care. *BMJ* 1993;**306**:1512–3.

4 Kerem E, Yatsiv I, Goitein K. Effect of endotracheal suctioning on arterial blood gases in children. *Int Care Med* 1990;**16**:95–9.

5 Dremers RR. Complications of endotracheal suctioning procedures. *Respiratory Care* 1982;**27**:453–7.

6 Simbruner G, Coradello H, Fodor M, *et al*. Effect of tracheal suction on oxygenation, circulation, and lung mechanics in newborn infants. *Arch Dis Child* 1981;**56**:326–30.

7 Skov L, Ryding J, Pryds O, Greisen G. Changes in cerebral oxygenation and cerebral blood volume during endotracheal suctioning in ventilated neonates. *Acta Paediatr* 1992;**81**:389–93.

8 Rasche RFH, Kuhns LR. Histopathologic changes in airway mucosa of infants after endotracheal intubation. *Pediatrics* 1972;**50**:632–7.

9 Fiorentini A. Potential hazards of tracheobronchial suctioning. *Inten Crit Care Nursing* 1992;**8**:217–26.

10 Hughes J, Gill A, Leach HJ, *et al*. A prospective study of the adverse effects of midazolam on withdrawal in critically ill children. *Acta Paediatr* 1994;**83**:1194–9.

11 Berde CB, Beyer JE, Bournaki M, *et al*. Comparison of morphine and methadone for prevention of postoperative pain in 3 to 7 year old children. *J Pediatr* 1991; **119**:136–41.

12 Anand KJS, Ingraham J. Tolerance, dependence and strategies for compassionate withdrawal of analgesics and anxiolytics in the paediatric ICU. *Critical Care Nurse* 1996;**16**:87–93.

13 Hoder EL, Leckman JF, Ehrenkranz R, *et al*. Clonidine in neonatal narcotic abstinence syndrome. *N Engl J Med* 1981;**305**:1284.

9 Management of long term pain and pain during terminal care

There are a number of situations in which children require control of long term pain. This may be during the course of a chronic disease, such as juvenile arthritis or sickle cell disease, or part of palliative care for a life-threatening illness such as progressive cancer or a neurodegenerative disorder.

It is important to remember that long term pain is different from acute pain in several ways. For example, verbal complaints tend to be less common. The child may become withdrawn, with decreased motor activity, less interest in play, a poor appetite, sleep disturbance and decreased concentration. Paradoxically, some children may play excessively to distract themselves from the pain. The child may become more and more difficult to console, and psychological issues tend to be more prominent: the child may be anxious or depressed, and frightened of his or her illness.

Common anxieties among sick children include:

- Concern that the treatment will be worse than the disease.
- Fear of hospital admission.
- Concern about the effect of the illness on their parents.
- Realisation that pain may reflect disease progression.

The severity of long term pain in children is easily underestimated, particularly by professionals.

MANAGEMENT OF LONG TERM PAIN

Important steps in the management of long term pain in a child are to assess the child, to formulate and implement a plan, and to reassess. Regular reassessment should include noting the level of pain relief, the presence of any side effects and the family's coping ability.

ASSESSMENT OF LONG TERM PAIN

Assessment of long term pain involves consideration of:

- The pain itself:
  — site: use body charts
  — nature: pain can be nocioceptive or neuropathic
  — severity: use age-appropriate objective tools (see pages 9–13 and Appendices A and B)
  — timing: use diaries (see Appendix C)
  — precipitating and relieving factors: use diaries.
- The child's and family's coping skills.
- The child's and family's past experiences of pain and coping strategies.
- The child's and family's anxiety and emotional distress.
- What the pain and the underlying disease mean to the child and family.

MANAGEMENT PLAN

When developing a management plan for the control of long term pain consider treatment directed at the underlying disease, for example, radiotherapy. Symptomatic treatment for the pain itself may be pharmacological or non-pharmacological or both (see earlier chapters).

A firm, therapeutic alliance should be established between patient, family and all of the professionals involved in caring for the child. Parents and child can be encouraged to share control of treatment and responsibility for its effectiveness. This may be achieved through:

- Explanation, reassurance, teaching and discussion.
- Establishing realistic short term and long term goals.
- Learning to incorporate distraction, relaxation and hypnosis where appropriate.
- Regular reassessment.
- Giving close attention to practical details, such as provision of aids for comfort.
- Considering the wider social and spiritual needs of the child and family including clear plans for parents and access to 24 h advice/support.

● Planning ahead to prevent crises. For examples, ensuring that a range of analgesic drugs are always available at home, having a syringe pump in the home ahead of time, and provision of an anticonvulsant at home if a fit is likely to occur as the disease progresses.

PHARMACOLOGICAL MANAGEMENT OF LONG TERM PAIN

Use the World Health Organisation (WHO) ladder of treatment[1] for a systematic approach to pain control.

Step 1

Non-opioid analgesic (for example, paracetamol, NSAID)
± adjuvants (antidepressants, anticonvulsants, steroids)

If pain persists or increases

Step 2

Weak opioid analgesic (for example, codeine)
± non-opioid analgesic
± adjuvant drugs

If pain persists or increases

Step 3

Strong opioid analgesic (for example, morphine, diamorphine)
± non-opioid analgesic
± adjuvant drugs

The WHO ladder is applicable to the management of long term pain arising from any cause. Drugs of similar efficacy should not be substituted if pain control becomes ineffective. Instead, move to the next rung of the ladder or add a drug of similar efficacy but with a different or complimentary action; for example, add an NSAID to paracetamol.

Unless pain is truly intermittent and not predictable (rare), then drugs given as part of this regimen should be administered regularly according to their duration of action.

PALLIATIVE CARE FOR CHILDREN WITH LIFE-THREATENING ILLNESS

A child and family have many and complex needs during the course of a life-threatening illness and in the final stage of the child's life. The physical and psychosocial problems will vary depending on the diagnosis, the time course of the illness and the individual family's approach. All aspects of the child and family's care need to be considered and pain is likely to be one problem within a much wider picture.

The sick child and family should be offered as much flexibility and choice in their care as possible. This includes where the child is cared for and dies. The majority prefer care to be centred around the home but the option of care in hospital or a children's hospice and the freedom to move between should always be available.

Good communication and coordination of all aspects of care throughout the illness, and also between home, hospital and respite services is important for the family. Establishing one member of the professional team, such as the paediatric oncology nurse specialist or paediatric community nurse (for examples the Macmillan and CLIC—cancer and leukaemia in childhood—paediatric oncology outreach nurses) as a keyworker can facilitate this.

Provision of palliative care services for children and their families varies widely in different localities and according to the illness. Recent guidelines for providing and purchasing of palliative care in children are available[2] which highlight families' needs and should help to improve access to care.

STRONG OPIOIDS FOR PALLIATIVE CARE

In some children, non-opioids or weak opioids are all that are needed for the control of pain.

The two main strong opioids used in children with chronic pain are morphine and diamorphine. Morphine is preferred for the oral route; diamorphine, which is more soluble in water, is more convenient for subcutaneous or intravenous injection. (Only 1·6 ml water is needed to dissolve 1 g diamorphine hydrochloride; 20 ml is required to dissolve 1 g of morphine sulphate.) Diamorphine is metabolised to morphine and does not have any intrinsic advantages.

Morphine is metabolised mainly in the liver to M3G (an inactive metabolite) and M6G (an active metabolite more potent than morphine itself). These metabolites are eliminated mainly through the kidneys.

Oral morphine is subject to first pass metabolism in the liver; plasma concentrations of morphine are therefore low and metabolite levels relatively high. The active metabolite M6G is therefore of particular importance after oral dosing.

Children rapidly eliminate the morphine metabolites. Rapid elimination is most marked in younger children (those aged under 9 years); as a result there are relatively lower M6G to morphine ratios in this group,[3] who may therefore need relatively higher doses to achieve pain relief.

While many patients may not need more than doubling of their morphine dose a few may need very high daily doses (sometimes grams per day) and the patients' morphine level should be increased as necessary to relieve their pain. Such high doses may be particularly important in children with a solid tumour that has compressed spinal nerve roots, nerve plexuses, large peripheral nerves or the spinal cord.[4]

Having commenced opioids in this situation, it is unusual for it to be possible to discontinue such drugs. However, if the cause of the pain is addressed, for example by radiotherapy, then opioids should be weaned carefully to avoid withdrawal (see pages 73–4).

Doses of strong opioids

The following starting doses are advised for children with pain not relieved by non-opioids or a weak opioid. The dosing convention for treating chronic pain is presented here as per 24 h.

Oral dose

Immediate release morphine   1·5–2 mg/kg/24 h. Administer as six divided doses, giving a double dose at bedtime to avoid night-time waking.

Controlled release morphine   2 mg/kg/24 h divided into two doses given at 12 h intervals (occasionally the total daily dose is more effective if given in three doses at 8 h intervals).

Breakthrough pain

Immediate release morphine (in doses as above) should always be available. It can be given as often as needed (e.g. every hour) although it will usually last for 3–4 h.

Titration of morphine dose

The morphine dose should be titrated against the level of pain. If frequent breakthrough medication is needed the total dose of morphine taken during the day (regular plus "breakthrough" doses) is assessed. This total daily dose becomes the prescription for the next 24 h. Regular review of daily doses allows them to be adjusted according to the amount of breakthrough medication given. Usually increments of 30–50% of the total daily dose are required.

Routes of administration

The oral (enteral) route is preferred whenever possible for the administration of strong opioids, sometimes involving the use of a nasogastric tube or gastrostomy, particularly when long term care is required. If a patient is unable to take drugs orally/enterally usually because of vomiting or a decreasing level of consciousness, the preferred routes are rectal and subcutaneous, or intravenous if a central line is in place. There is no role for intramuscular injections, and in children with thrombocytopenia they can be particularly harmful.

A continuous 24 h infusion provides a steady level of analgesia and is preferred to intermittent doses. Simple infusion pumps (for example, the Graseby) are most convenient, especially for families using them at home. Transdermal patches of fentanyl are currently being investigated in this context.

Transferring to different routes of opioid administration

Oral morphine to subcutaneous diamorphine The potency of diamorphine by injection is approximately three times that of oral morphine. Therefore use one-third of the total daily oral morphine dose (in milligrams) of diamorphine over 24 h by infusion; for example, if a patient is receiving 60 mg MST Continus orally twice daily, the total 24 h dose is 120 mg. The equivalent total 24 h dose of diamorphine subcutaneously is 40 mg.

Oral morphine to subcutaneous morphine The potency of morphine by injection is approximately twice that of oral morphine. Therefore use one-half of the total daily oral morphine dose (in milligrams) of morphine over 24 h by infusion.

Oral morphine to rectal morphine Use the same doses in this case. Immediate release morphine is available as suppositories for use every 4 h. Slow release tablets can be given rectally, for use 12 hourly.

Side effects of strong opioids The active management of uncommon unpleasant side effects is important. However, the rigorous monitoring of vital signs that is necessary after surgery is not appropriate in palliative care. Pain relief is the main priority. The possibility of side effects should be explained to parents together with the methods for dealing with them. Children on strong opioids should be regularly assessed.

- Constipation is the main continuing side effect, so laxatives should always be given prophylactically (see page 29).
- The daytime drowsiness, dizziness and mental clouding that usually occur at the start of treatment, almost always resolve within a few days.

- Cognitive and psychomotor disturbances are minimal once patients are receiving a stable dose of opioid.
- Nausea and vomiting is rare in children as a result of morphine. When it does occur, it usually resolves within 2–3 days.
- Pruritus caused by opioids usually wears off, but antihistamines can be effective if it does not.
- Nightmares may occur. If they do, try haloperidol at night (50–100 microgram/kg).
- Hallucinations occur rarely, and again haloperidol (25–100 microgram/kg/24 h) may be helpful.
- Respiratory depression is rare in the conscious patient with chronic pain.
- Urinary retention may be a problem, especially after rapid dose escalation. Most children respond to measures such as a hot bath, warm packs or relief of constipation, but catheterisation may be required, usually temporarily.

USE OF NSAIDs

NSAIDs (see page 17) are especially good for pain with an inflammatory component and for bone pain, for example, diclofenac, either orally, via gastrostomy or as suppositories. They need to be used with care in children who are thrombocytopenic.

USE OF STEROIDS

Although steroids are commonly used in adult palliative care, in children the disadvantages often outweigh the advantages and their use is more controversial. Rapid weight gain, change in appearance and body image, violent mood swings and behaviour changes are common and distressing to both the children and families. Initial symptom relief is rarely maintained for long as the tumour progresses and a spiral of increasing doses and side effects can develop.

Situations where they may have a role are in reducing pain by reducing oedema around tumours which are compressing nerves or as a short course to relieve symptoms from a brain tumour or during a last important holiday. Dexamethasone 250–1000 microgram/kg/24 h in 2 or 3 divided doses can be used.

USE OF RADIOTHERAPY

Radiotherapy can be particularly helpful in treating isolated sites of disease if a tumour is radiosensitive. These may include bony metastases, relieving nerve compression by a solid tumour and isolated cerebral metastases. Single treatments or very short courses are often appropriate in palliative care.

SOME OTHER TYPES OF PAIN OR DISCOMFORT THAT CAN OCCUR IN TERMINALLY ILL CHILDREN

Gastrointestinal pain

The pain of bowel colic can be reduced by using loperamide (capsules 2 mg; syrup 2 mg in 10 ml):

1–2 years	250–500 microgram	2–3 times/24 h
2–5 years	1 mg	3–4 times/24 h
6–12 years	2 mg	3–4 times/24 h

or hyoscine butylbromide (Buscopan) (tablets: 10 mg):

Under 6 years	5 mg	2–3 times/24 h
Over 6 years	10 mg	2–3 times/24 h

Hyoscine butylbromide can also be given as a subcutaneous or intravenous infusion in a dose of:

Under 6 years	15 mg/24 h
Over 6 years	15–30 mg/24 h

Headaches

Although headaches due to raised intracranial pressure may respond temporarily to high doses of dexamethasone (500 microgram/kg/24 h for 5 days then if possible reducing to 125 to 250 microgram/kg/24 h thereafter) a spiral of increasing and long term steroids should be avoided. Analgesics can be used according to the WHO classification. Headaches from meningeal leukaemia respond well to intrathecal chemotherapy.

Dyspnoea

Any reversible causes should be treated (for example, bronchospasm). The sensation of breathlessness can be relieved by oral or systemic opioids. The addition of diazepam to reduce anxiety (see page 75) may be helpful. Oxygen is rarely helpful for children with cancer but may be useful for those with chronic progressive lung disease, relieving headaches and improving sleep.

Intractable cough

If not prevented by the use of oral morphine or systemic diamorphine, this may be helped by moist inhalations such as:

Menthol and eucalyptus inhalation BP 1980 (1 teaspoon to a pint of hot (not boiling) water for inhalation) or Karvol capsules (1 capsule into a pint of hot (not boiling) water for inhalation).

Excessive respiratory secretions

These may be reduced by the use of hyoscine hydrobromide. (This is not the same drug as hyoscine butylbromide described above.) Hyoscine hydrobromide, can be given orally or by continuous subcutaneous infusion orally:

1–4 years	10 microgram/kg per dose every 6 h
5–12 years	10 microgram/kg per dose to a maximum of 400 microgram every 6 h
Over 12 years	400 microgram per dose every 6 h

By infusion use the total daily oral dose over 24 h.

Insomnia

Insomnia may be related to the presence of pain or the fear about the illness and death. These should be considered before sedation. If the child continues to be unable to sleep, benzodiazepines such as temazepam 0·5–1 mg/kg at night may be helpful. (Tablets 10 mg, elixir 10 mg in 5 ml.)

Neuropathic pain

Neuropathic pain, which is generally due to nerve infiltration or compression, is only partially responsive to opioids. It should be considered particularly if the pain has an unusual nature, for example burning or shooting. Two classes of drugs are valuable and should be started early on if possible:

Tricyclic antidepressants

Tricyclic antidepressants such as amitriptyline may be helpful, especially in treating the burning pain caused by nerve compression, invasion by tumour or from neuropathy (for example, that caused by vincristine). The starting dose of amitriptyline is 500 microgram/kg at night (increasing if needed to 1 mg/kg twice daily).

Anticonvulsants

Anticonvulsants such as carbamazepine may be helpful, especially when neuropathic pain is shooting or stabbing. Start with a low dose of 2·5 mg/kg twice a day, and increase gradually by 2·5–5 mg/kg/day at weekly intervals. The usual maintenance dose is 10–20 mg/kg/24 h (consider using controlled release tablets). Therapeutic blood levels range from 4–14 mg/l.

Nerve blocks may be helpful when pain is limited to a specific area. Transcutaneous electrical nerve stimulation (TENS) may also provide useful relief, but needs further evaluation.

USE OF MUSCLE RELAXANTS

Muscle spasm can be severe in central nervous system disease and is particularly common in children with neurodegenerative diseases. While muscle spasm occurs spontaneously and is painful and distressing in itself, it can also be triggered by pain elsewhere, for example, toothache, constipation, oral thrush, and attention to other pains may give relief of spasm.

Diazepam

Start with 100 microgram/kg diazepam every 6–12 h and titrate for effect. High doses are sometimes necessary but unacceptable drowsiness may limit the drug's efficacy. For acute exacerbations, rectal diazepam (e.g. Stesolid) may be necessary at anticonvulsant doses.

Baclofen

Preparations available: 10 mg tablets and 5 mg/5 ml syrup.

Start with 0·75–2 mg/kg/24 h baclofen, increasing every 2 days until control is achieved. Usual maximum total daily doses are: age 1–5 years, 30 mg/24 h; age 6–8 years, 40 mg/24 h; age 9–12 years, 60 mg/24 h; age 13–16 years, 100 mg/24 h. Doses are given on a three times a day basis.[5] It should be used with caution in renal impairment.

Combinations of diazepam and baclofen may give relief when either alone is ineffective.

LOCAL AND REGIONAL ANAESTHETICS

If there is persistent and localised pain, as from a joint in rheumatic disorders, injecting a local anaesthetic may provide short term relief. Occasionally an epidural or coeliac plexus block may provide short term relief for localised, intractable pain from malignancy.

USE OF SEDATIVES IN PALLIATIVE CARE

If anxiety is a major problem, attempts should be made to seek out the source. It may be related to a particular symptom, for example, dyspnoea and this can be treated. Often it is related to fear and concerns about the illness and its progression and this should be addressed through age-appropriate discussion or play.

Sometimes anxiety can reflect depression and under these circumstances an antidepressant (for example, amitriptyline) may help. Diazepam may also be helpful if anxiety persists.

Sedation may also be helpful in the final stages of a child's illness to relieve terminal agitation and distress. When used as a continuous infusion the following may be valuable in addition to diamorphine:

- Midazolam (sedating anticonvulsant and anxiolytic).
- Methotrimeprazine (sedating and anti-emetic).
- Haloperidol (sedating and anti-emetic).

MIXING AND COMPATIBILITY OF DRUGS

The general principle that injections should be given into separate sites and should not be mixed does not apply to the use of syringe pumps in palliative care.

The following drugs can be mixed with diamorphine as part of continuous subcutaneous or intravenous infusions:

- Cyclizine. However, cyclizine may precipitate at concentrations above 10 mg/ml, or in the presence of physiological saline, or as the concentrations of diamorphine relative to cyclizine increases. Mixtures of diamorphine and cyclizine are also liable to precipitate after being mixed for 24 h or more.
- Dexamethasone—special care is needed to avoid precipitation of dexamethasone when preparing the solution.
- Haloperidol—mixtures of haloperidol and diamorphine are liable to precipitate after 24 h if the haloperidol concentration is above 2 mg/ml.
- Hyoscine butylbromide.
- Hyoscine hydrobromide.
- Metoclopramide or methotrimeprazine.
- Midazolam.

Subcutaneous infusion solutions should be monitored regularly both to check for precipitation and discoloration and to ensure that the infusion is running at the correct rate.

Chlorpromazine, prochlorperazine and diazepam are contra-indicated subcutaneously as they cause skin reactions at the injection site. They can be given intravenously as a continuous infusion, ideally into an existing central line.

Diamorphine can be given by subcutaneous infusion at a strength of up to 250 mg/ml. When used in a concentration of up to 40 mg/ml either "water for injection" or 0·9% saline are suitable diluents. Above that strength, that is from 50 mg/ml–250 mg/ml only "water for injection" should be used to avoid precipitation.

Injections dissolved in "water for injection" are more likely to be associated with pain (possibly due to their hypotonicity). The use of physiological saline (sodium chloride 0·9%), however, increases the likelihood of precipitation when more than one drug is used. However, when low rates of subcutaneous infusion are used (for example, 0·1–0·3 ml/h) pain is not usually a problem when water is used as a diluent.

USE OF SYRINGE DRIVERS (SUBCUTANEOUS AND INTRAVENOUS)

- Local anaesthetic cream can be used to avoid anxiety and pain for the child when the subcutaneous needle is inserted.
- If the infusion runs too quickly check the rate setting in the calculation.
- If the infusion runs too slowly check the start button, the battery, the syringe driver and the cannula and make sure that the injection site is not inflamed.
- If there is an injection site reaction during subcutaneous infusion make sure that the site does not need to be changed—firmness or swelling at the site of injection is not in itself an indication of the change but pain and obvious inflammation is.
- When using intravenous infusions through central lines, luer locks should be used and the syringe should be placed below the level of the heart to avoid syphoning.
- Syringe drivers can be carried around by patients. They should not automatically mean that a child is confined to the home.

It should be noted from the above that non-licensed indications or routes are being recommended for use in palliative care.

REFERENCES

1 World Health Organisation. *Cancer pain relief and palliative care* (Technical Report Series 804). Geneva:WHO, 1990.
2 Report of joint working parties of The Association for Children with Life-threatening or Terminal Conditions and their Families and the Royal College of Paediatrics and Child Health. *A guide to the development of children's palliative care services.* RCPCH, London, 1997.
3 Hunt A, Joel S, Gloyn A, Goldman A. Pharmacokinetics of immediate-release oral morphine liquid and its glucuronides in children with cancer pain. *Eur J Pall Care.* Abstracts of the Fourth Congress of the European Association for Palliative Care, 6–9 December 1995, Barcelona, Spain.
4 Collins JJ, Grier HE, Kinney HC, Berde CB. Control of severe pain in children with terminal malignancy. *J Pediatr* 1995;**126**:653–7.
5 Brady M. Symptom control in dying children. In: Hill L. *Caring for dying children and their families.* London: Chapman & Hall, 1994;123–61.

10 Managing pain in sickle cell disease

Unlike cancer pain, pain from sickle cell disease is intermittent and time limited. As yet, we have no objective marker to distinguish vaso-occlusive pain from other pain. Management of pain in sickle cell disease[1] requires an understanding of the complex mixture of acute and chronic aspects of the disease, and support of the whole child's needs within the family.[2]

The approach to pain control should be stepwise (see page 80), and pharmacological and non-pharmacological approaches are required.

Written agreements, involving the patient, family and health professionals should be provided. These are especially valuable in adolescents who undergo frequent hospital admissions for pain. Agreements should be changed only by mutual consent of all involved in drawing up the document, and include treatment plans for home use (Appendix G).

Interrupted school attendance may cause serious educational difficulties for children with sickle cell disease. Liaise with the school and advocate extra tuition.

PHARMACOLOGICAL MANAGEMENT

Episodes of severe pain may require very large opioid doses. Doses of intravenous or subcutaneous morphine higher than those used postoperatively may be needed (average 100 microgram/kg/h, maximum 400 microgram/kg/h).[3]

Start treatment as soon as possible, before the pain becomes a problem. Sometimes it might be difficult to find a vein and if an intravenous cannula is difficult to site, a single intramuscular injection may have to be used to avoid delay in initiating analgesia.

Considerable individualisation of the doses of morphine may be required to achieve optimal analgesia with minimum side effects.[4] Intravenous methylprednisolone has been recently reported to reduce the duration of opioid treatment required to control pain.[5]

Inpatient care

Take care that respiratory depression does not produce atelectasis and a reduction in arterial oxygenation, as this may increase sickling. Monitor oxygen saturation.

Patient controlled analgesia (see page 25) is valuable in the early stages of a vaso-occlusive episode.

Patients should be weaned from strong opioids using decreasing doses rather than increasing intervals. Proceed slowly, to avoid the need to backtrack. There is no fixed formula: use the WHO ladder in reverse (see page 80). Do not use "prn" doses, as this may increase the risk of drug misuse.

Epidural analgesia containing local anaesthetics with or without fentanyl may safely treat pain unresponsive to intravenous opioids without causing sedation, respiratory depression or significant limitation of movement. It may also improve oxygenation.[6]

NON-PHARMACOLOGICAL MANAGEMENT

As when managing chronic pain, include the child and his or her family in discussions concerning pain control.

Ensure adequate hydration (give fluids 125–150% of maintenance) and give oxygen if oxygen saturation falls below 95%.

Apply chest physiotherapy and deep breathing exercises. Give red cell transfusions only for life-threatening problems like progressive acute chest syndrome. The latter is more likely if there has been insufficient analgesia given.

TENS[7] and hypnosis (see page 37) may be valuable. Heat packs/hot baths/splints may be helpful for sickling that involves peripheral joints.

CARE IN THE ACCIDENT AND EMERGENCY DEPARTMENT

Keep the patient's written agreement available. Respect the patient's knowledge of previous drugs and doses that have worked, and contact the patient's own consultant as soon as possible.

REFERENCES

1 Grundy R, Howard R, Evans J. Practical management of pain in sickling disorders. *Arch Dis Child* 1993;**69**:256–9.

2 Shapiro BS, Dinges DF, Orne EC, *et al.* Home management of sickle cell related pain in infants and adolescents: natural history and impact on school attendance. *Pain* 1995;**61**:139–44.

3 Shapiro BS. Management of painful episodes in sickle cell disease. In: Schecheter NL, Berde CB, Yaster, M. eds. *Pain in infants, children and adolescents.* Williams & Wilkins: Baltimore, 1992.

4 Dampier CD, Setty BNY, Logan J, *et al.* Intravenous morphine pharmacokinetics in pediatric patients with sickle cell disease. *J Pediatr* 1995;**126**:461–7.

5 Griffin TC, McIntire D, Buchanan GR. High dose intravenous methylprednisolone therapy for pain in children and adolescents with sickle cell disease. *N Engl J Med* 1994;**330**:733–7.

6 Yaster M, Tobin JR, Billett C, *et al.* Epidural analgesia in the management of severe vaso-occlusive sickle cell crisis. *Pediatrics* 1994;**93**:310–5.

7 Lander J, Fowler-Kerry S. TENS for children's procedural pain. *Pain* 1993;**52**:209–16.

11 Further reading and resources

FURTHER READING

ABPI *Data sheet compendium* 1995–6. ISBN 090710207. London: Datapham Publications Ltd.

Report of a joint ACT/Royal College of Paediatrics and Child Health Working Party. *A Guide to the Development of Children's Palliative Care Services*. London: RCPCH, 1997.

The Northern Neonatal Network, *Neonatal formulary*. London: BMJ Publishing Group, 1996.

Alder Hey book of children's doses. Liverpool, Alder Hey Children's Hospital, 1994.

Paediatric formulary. (3rd ed). London: Guy's, Lewisham and St Thomas's Hospitals. London: British Medical Association, 1993.

Neonatal formulary. London: Hammersmith and Queen Charlotte's Hospitals, 1993.

British national formulary. London: British Medical Association, 1996.

Consumers' Association. Treating moderate and severe pain in infants. *Drug Ther Bull* 1994;**32**:21–4.

McCaffery M, Beebe A. *Pain: clinical manual for nursing practice*. St Louis: CV Mosby, 1989.

The RVI book of acute pain management in children. Newcastle upon Tyne: Royal Victoria Infirmary, 1994.

Drug administration guidelines. Department of Anaesthesia Acute Pain Service, Great Ormond Street Hospital for Children NHS Trust. London, 1996 (4th ed).

Schechter NL, Berde CB, Yaster M. *Pain in infants, children and adolescents*. Baltimore: Williams & Wilkins, 1992.

Lloyd-Thomas AR. Pain management in paediatric patients. *Br J Anaesth* 1990;**64**:85–104.

Lloyd-Thomas AR, Howard RF. A pain service for children. *Paediatr Anaesth* 1994;**4**:3–15.

Lloyd-Thomas AR. Post-operative pain control in children. *Curr Paediatr* 1993;**3**:234–7.

Burr S. Pain in childhood. *Nursing* 1987;**24**:890–5.

Goldman A. Pain management. *Arch Dis Child* 1993;**68**:423–5.

Russell SCS, Doyle E. Recent advances in paediatric anaesthesia. *BMJ* 1997;**314**:201–3.

Walco GA, Cassidy RC, Schechter NL. Pain, hurt, and harm. The ethics of pain control in infants and children. *N Engl J Med* 1994;**331**:541–4.

Cote CJ. Sedation for the pediatric patient: a review. *Pediatr Clin North Am* 1994;**41**:31–58.

Tyler DC. Pharmacology of pain management. *Pediatr Clin North Am* 1994;**41**:59–71.

Fitzgerald M. Developmental biology of inflammatory pain. *Br J Anaesth* 1995;**75**:177–85.

Lloyd-Thomas AR. Assessment and control of pain in children. *Anaesthesia* 1995;**50**:753–5.

Consumers' Association. Managing acute pain in children. *Drug Ther Bull* 1995;**33**:41–4.

Hill L, ed. *Caring for dying children and their families.* London: Chapman & Hall, 1994.

Ainsley Green A, Ward Platt MP, Lloyd-Thomas AR. Stress and pain in infancy and childhood. *Baillière's Clinical Paediatrics* 1995; **3**(3).

RESOURCES

Booklets

- *Children and pain.* Available from: Action for Sick Children, Argyle House, 29–31 Euston Road, London NW1 2SD.
- *Needles. Helping to take away the fear.* Available from: Action for Sick Children, Argyle House, 29–31 Euston Road, London NW1 2SD.
- *RCN standards of care project 1994* (for the assessment of pain/physical discomfort). Available from: Royal College of Nursing of the UK, Viking House, 17–19 Peterborough Road, Harrow, Middlesex HA1 2AX.

Videos

- *Patient controlled analgesia.* Available from: Department of Medical Photography, Royal Liverpool Children's NHS Trust, Alder Hey, Eaton Road, Liverpool L12 2AP; Tel: 0151–228 4811 ext. 2283/ 3013.
- *Painful procedures—helping children to cope.* Available from: Trust Fund 21/204, PALS, c/o Paediatric Renal Unit, City Hospital, Hucknall Road, Nottingham NG5 1PB.
- *No tears, no fears: children with cancer coping with pain.* Canadian Cancer Society, 955 W Broadway, Vancouver, BC V5X 3X8, Canada.

Complementary therapy unit for children

At the Queen's Medical Centre in Nottingham, one of the first complementary therapy services has been set up for children. Clinics are held on a regular basis, offering relaxation therapy/ techniques, therapeutic touch, massage and aromatherapy. They are offered to all children with a variety of conditions, including those suffering from long term pain.

Complementary therapy is used, in conjunction with orthodox medical and nursing treatments, to enhance patient wellbeing, quality of life and to provide symptomatic relief.

Massage can be used to relieve postchemotherapy side effects, for example, aching muscles following a course of vincristine.

Relaxation techniques involving music and an aromatherapy burner can help to relieve anxiety which can make symptoms of certain illness worse. Parents are taught how to use the techniques so that they can apply them to their children.

Sources of advice on hypnosis

British Hypnosis Research
Southpoint
8 Paston Place
Brighton BN2 1HA

Tel: (01273) 693 622

British Hypnotherapy Association
1 Wythburn Place
London W1H 5WI

Tel: (0171) 262 8852/723 4443

British Society of Medical and
Dental Hypnosis
48 Links Road
Ashtead
Surrey KT31 3JH

Tel: (01372) 273 522

National College for Hypnotherapy
and Psychotherapy
12 Cross Street
Nelson
Lancashire BB9 7EN

Owl College of Hypnosis
2 Buchanan Street
Leigh
Greater Manchester WN7 1XT

Therapy Training College
8–10 Balaclava Street
Kings Heath
Birmingham B14 7SG

Tel: (0121) 444 5435

UK Training College of
Hypnotherapy and Counselling
10 Alexander Street
London W2 5NT

Tel: (0171) 221 1796/727 2006

World Federation of
Hypnotherapists
Belmont Square
Ramsgate
Kent CT11 7QG

Tel: (01843) 587 929

Appendix A Self report scales for pain assessment

Measure	Description	Indications for use	Advantages	Disadvantages
Self report measure	Child is asked re. intensity, rhythm and variations in pain	Adequate cognitive and communicative abilities	Simple, efficient, easily administered	Subject to bias (e.g. demand characteristics, inaccurate or selective memory)
Poker Chip Tool Available from: Dr N Hester School of Nursing, C288 University of Colorado Health Sciences Centre, 4200 East Ninth Avenue, Denver, CO 80262	Child chooses 1–4 chips (chips = "piece of hurt")	Age 4–8 years	Correlates with overt behaviours during injections; adequate convergent validity; partial support for discriminant validity	May seem childish to older children
Faces scale[4]	Faces indicating pain intensity were derived from children's drawings	Age 6–8 years	Strong agreement among children re. pain severity of faces and consistency of intervals. Adequate test–retest reliability	Younger child may tend to choose happiest face; may also choose extremes
Visual analogue scale[5]	Vertical or horizontal line with verbal, facial or numerical anchors on a continuum of pain intensity	Age 5 years and over	Reliable and valid (child report correlates with behavioural measures and with parent, nurse, physician ratings). Versatile (can rate different dimensions—pain and affect—on same scale)	Child must understand proportionality. Intervals on numerical scales may not be equal from a child's perspective. Vertical scale may be better than horizontal.

(continued)

Measure	Description	Indications for use	Advantages	Disadvantages
Oucher scale[6]	Six photos of children's faces indicating intensity; 100-point corresponding vertical scale	Age 3–12 years	Reliable; adequate content validity; correlates with other scales. Pictorial plus numerical scales, so applicable to broader age range	See Visual Analogue Scale

Other scales:

- Eland Colour Tool,[7] available from Dr J. Eland, 316 Nursing, University of Iowa, Iowa City, IA 52242
- Varni Thompson Pediatric Pain Questionnaire,[8] available from Dr J.W. Varni, Behavioural Pediatrics Program, Orthopaedic Hospital, 2400 South Flower Street, Los Angeles, CA 90007
- Adolescent Pediatric Pain Tool,[9] available from Dr M Savedra, University of California at San Francisco, School of Nursing, San Francisco CA 94143-0606
- Children's Pain Inventory,[10] available from Dr P.A. McGrath, Department of Pediatrics, Children's Hospital of Western Ontario, London, Ontario, Canada N6C 2V5

For references see page 13.

Appendix B   Behavioural scales for pain assessment

Measure	Description	Indications for use	Advantages	Disadvantages
Behavioural measures	Direct observation of overt behaviours, usually measured repeatedly at regular intervals, according to time or phase of procedure	Very young children. Used with self report scale. Best reliability and validity are for short, sharp pain	Useful when child is unable to rate pain; less subject to bias than self report	Not as well validated for longer lasting pain or for subtle behaviours (e.g. guarding wound). Difficult to discriminate
Procedural rating scale[11] and observational scale of behavioural distress[12] (OSBD)	10 observed behaviours: crying, screaming, need for physical restraint, verbal resistance, requests for emotional support, muscular rigidity, verbal pain expression, flailing, nervous behaviour, information-seeking	Originally used for bone marrow aspiration and lumbar puncture, but appropriate for any short, sharp pain	Satisfactory inter-rater reliability; OSBD correlates with self report of pain and anxiety	Requires training of observers
Children's Hospital of Eastern Ontario pain scale (CHEOPS)[13]	Six observed behaviours: crying, facial expression, verbal expression, torso position, leg position, touch	Originally used for postoperative pain and needle pain	Easy to learn and use. Inter-rater reliability = 80% concurrent validity	Insensitive to long term pain
Gauvain-Piquard rating scale 14	15 behaviours divided into three subscales: pain behaviours (e.g. guarding wound), anxiety behaviours (e.g. nervousness), psychomotor alterations (e.g. withdrawal)	Validated with 2–6 year olds. Used for long term pain in children with cancer	Preliminary studies show adequate inter-rater reliability and sensitivity to differences in children	Validity studies not yet completed

Behavioural definitions and scoring of the CHEOPS scale to measure postoperative pain

Item	Behaviour	Score	Definition
Cry	No cry	1	Child is not crying
	Moaning	2	Child is moaning or quietly vocalising; silent cry
	Crying	2	Child is crying, but the cry is gentle or whimpering
	Scream	3	Child is in a full-lunged cry; sobbing; may be scored with complaint or without complaint
Facial	Composed	1	Neutral facial expression
	Grimace	2	Score only if definite negative facial expression
	Smiling	0	Score only if definite positive facial expression
Child verbal	None	1	Child not talking
	Other complaints	1	Child complains, but not about pain; e.g. "I want to see Mummy" or "I am thirsty"
	Pain complaints	2	Child complains about pain
	Both complaints	2	Child complains about pain and about other things; e.g. "It hurts; I want Mummy"
	Positive	0	Child makes any positive statement or talks about other things without complaint
Torso	Neutral	1	Body (not limbs) is at rest; torso is inactive
	Shifting	2	Body is in motion in a shifting or serpentine fashion
	Tense	2	Body is arched or rigid
	Shivering	2	Body is shuddering or shaking involuntarily
	Upright	2	Child is in vertical or upright position
	Restrained	2	Body is restrained
Touch	Not touching	1	Child is not touching or grabbing at wound
	Reach	2	Child is reaching for but not touching wound
	Touch	2	Child is gently touching wound or wound area
	Grab	2	Child is grabbing vigorously at wound
	Restrained	2	Child's arms are restrained
Legs	Neutral	1	Legs may be in any position but are relaxed; includes gentle swimming or serpentine-like movements
	Squirming/kicking	2	Definitive uneasy or restless movements in the legs and/or striking out with foot or feet
	Drawn up/tensed	2	Legs tensed and/or pulled up tightly to body and kept there
	Standing	2	Standing, crouching or kneeling
	Restrained	2	Child's legs are being held down

From McGrath PJ, *et al*. The CHEOPS: a behavioural scale to measure postoperative pain in children. In: Fields HL, Dubner R, Cervero R, eds. *Advances in pain research and therapy*. New York: Raven Press, 1985.

Appendix C   Diary for pain assessment

1 ⊢————————————————————⊣ 10

Visual Analogue Scale with numerical anchors

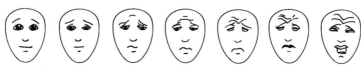

Faces Scale

INSTRUCTIONS FOR THE DIARY

1. Be sure to fill out your own diary at breakfast, lunch, dinner and bedtime each day. If you forget to record at one of these times, draw a line through that space.

2. Fill in the diary for how you are at the time.

3. **Severity of pain:** Use the numbers from the severity of pain chart at the bottom of the page to show how you are at the time. Be sure to mark a "0" if you have no pain.

4. **Other symptoms:** Write in anything else you feel at this time, such as nausea, vomiting, dizziness, visual disturbance, loss of appetite, etc. If you feel nothing else draw a line through the space.

5. **Medication:** Please write in the name and amount of any medication you have taken since the last period. If none was taken, please draw a line through that space.

6. **Possible cause:** Write in anything you think might have caused the pain, such as a change in the weather, an exam, an argument with parents or friends, a particular food, an allergy, etc. If you do not know draw a line through the space.

7. **Exercise:** Please write down at what time you did your relaxation exercise for each day.

Faces Scale: reproduced from Bieri, *et al.* (see reference 4 in Chapter 2) with permission from the authors and publishers.

Fill in this form at breakfast, lunch, dinner and bedtime each day

Name: _____ Week beginning: _____

Day	Time	Severity of pain	Other symptoms	Medication	Possible cause
	Breakfast				
	Lunch				
	Dinner				
	Bedtime				
	Breakfast				
	Lunch				
	Dinner				
	Bedtime				
	Breakfast				
	Lunch				
	Dinner				
	Bedtime				
	Breakfast				
	Lunch				
	Dinner				
	Bedtime				
	Breakfast				
	Lunch				
	Dinner				
	Bedtime				
	Breakfast				
	Lunch				
	Dinner				
	Bedtime				
	Breakfast				
	Lunch				
	Dinner				
	Bedtime				

Severity of pain

0 – No pain

1 – Pain – I am only aware of it if I pay attention to it

2 – Pain – but I can ignore it at times

3 – Pain – I can't ignore it, but I can do my usual activities

4 – Pain – It is difficult for me to concentrate; I can only do easy activities

5 – Pain – such that I can't do anything

Pain diary

Pain Diary: modified from McGrath P, *et al. Help yourself: a treatment for migraine headaches.* Ottawa: University of Ottawa Press, 1990.

Appendix D   Sample charts for monitoring pain control

Any problems Monday to Friday 0830–1700: contact Clinical Nurse Specialist, Pain Relief: page –ext.–

Epidural Protocol

Serial no. of pump ....

Signature of anaesthetist ....

Date & time started ....

Name .... Unit no .... D.o.B. .... Age .... Weight ....

Operation.. Date ....

Epidural site Thoracic Lumbar Caudal   1 2 3 4 5 6 7 8 9 10 11 12

Needle size   16G   18G   19G

Length of catheter in epidural space   cm   Mark on skin   cm

Prescription

In theatre	Bupivacaine	0.5%	0.25%	0.125%	0.166%	vol ml
In recovery	Bupivacaine	0.5%	0.25%	0.125%	0.166%	vol ml
Infusion	Bupivacaine	0.125%	0.166%	at ____ to ____		ml/h
Top-ups	Bupivacaine	0.25%	_____ml			

Max dose per 4 h 1.25–1.5 mg/kg if < 6 months; 2 mg/kg if 6 months or older = ☐ **mg per 4 h**

Record hourly (AFTER TOP-UPS record every 5 min for 15 min)

Time	Spo₂	RR	BP sys/ dia	HR	Height of block	SEDATION SCORE Eyes open: 0=spontaneously 1=to speech 2=to shake **3=unrousable** **(call doctor)**	PAIN SCORE at rest Eyes open: 0=no pain A=asleep 1=not really sore 2=quite sore **3=very sore** **(crying)** **(call doctor)**	NAUSEA SCORE 0=none 1=nausea only 2=vomiting x 1 in last hour **3=vomiting** >1 in last hour **(call doctor)**	RESTLESSNESS SCORE 0=none 1=slight (easily calmed) 2=moderate (not easily calmed) **3=severe** **(inconsolable, may need to top up sedation)** **(call doctor)**	RECORD TOP-UPS as volume conc sedation as drug, mg, route, time	Volume left in syringe (ml)

CALL DOCTOR if: pain score 3; nausea score 3; restlessness score 3; syringe empty

CONTACT DOCTOR AND SWITCH OFF EPIDURAL if patient unrousable (score 3); Spo₂<95%

block height above ☐   HR< ☐   BP< ☐

CONTACT duty anaesthetist bleep if help needed, or Dr............................. Home no.....................

102

Any problems Monday to Friday 0830–1700: contact Clinical Nurse Specialist, Pain Relief: page–ext.–

Intravenous Morphine Infusion
(Please place completed chart in casenotes)

Name .... Unit no .... D.o.B. .... Age .... Weight ....

Operation .... Date ....

Morphine concentration (1 mg/kg in 50 ml 0·9% saline) .... (maximum 50 mg in 50 ml)

Rate from .... ml/h to .... ml/h

Any adjustments (specify type, reason and time made) ....

> *Serial no. of pump* ....
>
> *Signature of anaesthetist* ....
>
> *Date & time infusion started* ....

Record hourly

Time	SpO₂	Resp rate	SEDATION SCORE Eyes open: 0 = spontaneously 1 = to speech 2 = to shake **3 = unrousable** **(call doctor)**	PAIN SCORE 0 = no pain A = asleep 1 = not really sore 2 = quite sore **3 = very sore** **(crying)** **(call doctor)**	NAUSEA SCORE 0 = none 1 = nausea only 2 = vomiting x 1 in last hour **3 = vomiting** **>1 in last hour** **(call doctor)**	Rate of infusion (ml/h)	Volume left in syringe

CALL DOCTOR if: severe pain (score 3); patient unrousable (sedation score 3); SpO₂<95%; respiration rate <10 min if over 5 years; <20 min if under 5 years; excessive nausea or vomiting; drip blocked/tissued or pump alarming. If patient unrousable, switch off pump and consider naloxone, 10 microgram/kg intravenously.

CONTACT duty anaesthetist if help needed, or Dr...................................... Home no ....

103

Any problems Monday to Friday 0830–1700: contact Clinical Nurse Specialist, Pain Relief: page –ext.–

PCA Protocol
(Please place completed chart in casenotes)

Name .... Unit no .... D.o.B. .... Age .... Weight ....

Operation .... Date ....

Morphine concentration (1 mg/kg in 50 ml 0.9% saline, i.e. 20 microgram/kg/ml) = ... mg/ml

(maximum 50 mg in 50 ml)

Bolus dose (20 microgram/kg) = ... mg (= 1 ml)

Lockout interval 5 min. Background infusion 0·2 ml/h (4 microgram/kg/h) = ... mg/h

Any adjustments (specify type, reason and time made) ....

Serial no. of pump ....
Signature of anaesthetist ....
Date & time infusion started ....

Record hourly

Time	SpO₂	Resp rate	SEDATION SCORE Eyes open: 0 = spontaneously 1 = to speech 2 = to shake 3 = unrousable (call doctor)	Pain score at rest 0 = no pain A = asleep 1 = not really sore 2 = quite sore 3 = very sore (crying) (call doctor)	Pain score on movement (deep breath in and cough)	NAUSEA SCORE 0 = none 1 = nausea only 2 = vomiting x 1 in last hour 3 = vomiting >1 in last hour (call doctor)	Total dose since reset	Number of presses and % good (press verify)	Volume left in syringe

CALL DOCTOR if: severe pain (score 3); patient unrousable (sedation score 3); SpO₂ <95%; respiration rate <10 min if over 5 years; <20 min if under 5 years; excessive nausea or vomiting; drip blocked/tissued or pump alarming. If patient unrousable, switch off pump and consider naloxone, 10 microgram/kg intravenously.

CONTACT duty anaesthetist bleep if help needed, or Dr .... Home no ....

Appendix E Patient leaflet: epidural anaesthesia

WHAT IS AN EPIDURAL?

This is a very effective method of pain relief. While your child is asleep under a general anaesthetic, a fine tube is put into his or her back, into an area called the "epidural space". This space contains nerves that send messages from the sore place to your child's brain when he or she is in pain. A needle is used to put the tube into your child's back and then is pulled out, leaving the tube in place. There will be sticky tape on your child's back to stop the tube falling out. Local anaesthetic is given through the tube into the epidural space to "block" the nerves and stop the pain messages being carried. This means that the area where your child has surgery is numb and less painful.

HOW IS THE LOCAL ANAESTHETIC GIVEN?

There are two ways that we give local anaesthetic in this hospital. The first is that your child may have a pump attached to the tube in his or her back. The pump is set by the anaesthetist to give a continuous suitable dose of the local anaesthetic via the tube. The other method is that your child will receive the medicine only when he or she starts to feel sore. This is called a "top-up". The anaesthetist will give the medicine via the tube by using a syringe and squeezing it slowly. The medicine may make your child's legs feel heavy and slightly numb—but don't worry, this is normal.

OBSERVING YOUR CHILD WITH AN EPIDURAL

The nurses in the ward will watch your child closely if he or she has an epidural. They will check every hour to see if your child is comfortable and that the epidural is working properly. They will also check the blood pressure, as sometimes an epidural can lower this slightly.

If your child is having pain relief by the "top-up" method, the nurses will check the blood pressure every 5 minutes for 15 minutes after the top-up is given. Your child will be lying down at this time so that the medicine is spread evenly and the right area is covered.

Your child will be seen two or three times a day by someone from the hospital's Pain Relief Service, to make sure that he or she is comfortable.

OTHER POINTS

If your child is having the "top-up" version of epidural pain relief, the medicine given can last any time from 4 hours to 12 hours. At night there is always an anaesthetist in the hospital "on call". It is his specialist job to look after the epidurals. However, he also has to be available for any emergency operations. If your child starts to feel sore and the anaesthetist is in the operating theatre, he may not be able to come to "top-up" your child straightaway. To solve this problem, your child will have a small plastic tube called a cannula put in his or her arm while they are in theatre. This will not hurt and the tube will be held in place by a small piece of tape. Through this tube the nurses can give some strong pain killing medicine (usually morphine). This will stop your child feeling sore until the anaesthetist is able to come to the ward and top up the epidural.

Before your child's epidural is stopped, he or she will be started on other pain killing medicine. Usually a syrup, tablets or suppositories that will be given regularly through the day.

I hope this answers any queries you may have about epidurals. If there is anything you would like to discuss, please ask to speak to the Clinical Nurse Specialist in Pain Relief.

Appendix F   Patient leaflet: morphine

QUESTIONS ABOUT MORPHINE

Questions and concerns about medicines used to control pain are normal. We hope that this handout will answer your questions about your child's pain relief. The medicines we use are safe and very effective. They will help your child recover more easily and quickly from his or her surgery. If you have questions that are not answered in this handout, please ask to speak to the Clinical Nurse Specialist in Pain Relief.

SOME COMMON QUESTIONS

- Is morphine too strong for children?
- Will my child become addicted to morphine?
- Will my child have unpleasant side effects from morphine?

WHY DO WE USE MORPHINE?

Your child may have some pain after certain surgical procedures. Morphine and some morphine-like medicines are some of the most effective treatments to control this pain. These medicines are very safe when used properly. Your child should be able to move or cough without discomfort. If your child is to have physiotherapy after surgery and has good pain control, the treatment will be much more effective. Recovery and healing should take place more quickly.

IS MORPHINE TOO STRONG?

The pain relief effects of morphine depend on the dose given. In this hospital the doses are worked out for each child according to his or her weight and age. The children are watched carefully by the nurses and doctors in the wards. Special charts are filled in every hour by the ward nurses. These charts check the dose of medicine that your child is receiving and how effective it is. As your child's pain gets less, he or she is given less medicine.

CAN MORPHINE FOR PAIN CONTROL CAUSE ADDICTION?

Your child will not become addicted to the morphine that he or she is given to control pain. Addiction does not occur, even if a child needs morphine for a long time.

WILL MY CHILD HAVE UNPLEASANT SIDE EFFECTS FROM MORPHINE?

Sometimes morphine may make your child feel slightly sick or itchy. These side effects can be reduced by:

- Adjusting the dose of morphine.
- Giving other medicines to treat the side effects such as anti-sickness medicine.

Over-sleepiness is rare and should not be confused with your child "catching up" on sleep that he or she may have lost if very unwell before surgery.

WILL MY CHILD BE SORE WHEN MORPHINE IS STOPPED?

We often give regular doses of milder pain relief medicines, such as paracetamol or diclofenac, at the same time as morphine. These can be given as a tablet, syrup or suppository. They can help us to use less morphine and to stop the morphine sooner. When morphine is stopped, these milder drugs are given in adequate amounts to keep pain well controlled.

Appendix G   Pain control in sickle cell disease

Agreement for the home management of pain from vaso-occlusive sickling in a child

Name .... **Date of Contract** ....

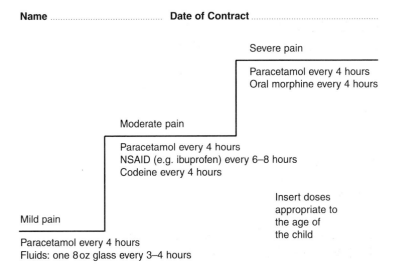

Severe pain

Paracetamol every 4 hours
Oral morphine every 4 hours

Moderate pain

Paracetamol every 4 hours
NSAID (e.g. ibuprofen) every 6–8 hours
Codeine every 4 hours

Insert doses
appropriate to
the age of
the child

Mild pain

Paracetamol every 4 hours
Fluids: one 8 oz glass every 3–4 hours

Go to the Accident and Emergency Department if:

- pain is not like the usual sickle cell pain
- vomiting prevents the taking of tablets
- medication has been given for 12 hours with no relief
- there is a fever (temperature above 101°F or 38°C)

Typical management of the above patient at the A&E department

- **Intravenous morphine** (loading dose 100–200 microgram/kg)
- Establish patient controlled analgesia
- If patient vomiting give intravenous fluids (125–150% maintenance)
- Establish diagnosis
- By regular assessment ensure pain is controlled adequately (may need very large doses of morphine)
- Monitor oxygen saturation: give O_2 if oxygen saturation is <95%
- Give appropriate laxatives to minimise the side effects of opioids
- Start non-pharmacological therapies
- Ensure sleep
- Wean from drugs carefully after 1–3 days

Index